**PHARMACEUTICAL
PRESS**
Essential Knowledge

Pharmacy Foundation Assessment Foundation 2

Pharmacy Foundation Assessment Questions 2

Sonia Kauser, MPharm, PGDip Hosp. Pharmacy, PGDip Advanced Practice, Independent Prescriber (Series Editor)
Advanced Clinical Pharmacist Practitioner, Lecturer in Pharmacy Practice / Assistant Professor Physician Associates

Cam Anh Tran Phan, MPharm, PGDip Clinical Pharmacy Secondary Care, PGCert Psychiatric Therapeutics, PracCert Independent Prescribing, PCPEP ExemptCert, FHEA, Celia Feetam Award Winner 2019 (Contributor)
Independent Prescribing Clinical Pharmacist at Porter Valley Primary Care Network (Sheffield), Assistant Professor in Pharmacy Practice at the University of Bradford and PhD candidate - National Institute for Health and Care Research (NIHR) Yorkshire and Humber Patient Safety Research Collaboration

Habib Shah, MPharm, MRPharmS, Independent Prescriber (Contributor)
Calderdale & Huddersfield NHS Foundation Trust Clinical Pharmacist PCN Trainee Pharmacist Programme, Co-lead Primary Healthcare Development Exams & Calculations lead, Senior PCN Clinical Pharmacist Trainee Pharmacist Designated Supervisor

Sadia Qayyum BSc Pharmacy (Hons), PGCert (Clinical Pharmacy), MRPharmS, SFHEA, Independent Prescriber (Contributor)
Lecturer in Pharmacy Practice (University of Manchester), Relief Manager (Well Pharmacy), GP Practice Pharmacist, Northern Lead for Primary Care Pharmacy Association

Misbah Noor Ansari, MPharm (Contributor)
Locum pharmacist

Shaheen Razzaq MPharm, PGCert Advanced Clinical Skills and Emergency Medicine, Independent Prescriber (Contributor)
Advanced Clinical Pharmacist Practitioner

Published by the Pharmaceutical Press

66-68 East Smithfield, London E1W 1AW
© Pharmaceutical Press 2025

PHARMACEUTICAL PRESS
Essential Knowledge

is a trade mark of Pharmaceutical Press. Pharmaceutical Press is the publishing division of the Royal Pharmaceutical Society.

First published 2025

Printed in Great Britain by TJ Books

ISBN 978-0-85711-466-2

All rights reserved. No part of this publication may be reproduced, stored in a retrieval system, or transmitted in any form or by any means, without the prior written permission of the copyright holder.

The publisher makes no representation, express or implied, with regard to the accuracy of the information contained in this book and cannot accept any legal responsibility or liability for any errors or omissions that may be made.

The rights of Sony Kauser be identified as the editor of this work have been asserted by them in accordance with the Copyright, Designs and Patents Act, 1988.

A catalogue record for this book is available from the British Library.

Disclaimer

The views expressed in this book are solely those of the author and do not necessarily reflect the views or policies of the Royal Pharmaceutical Society. This book does NOT guarantee success in the registration exam but can be used as an aid for revision.

*Dedicated to my parents,
Mohammed Rayaz and Abida Bi.*

*With special thanks to Mark Pollard
for his review and guidance.*

Contents

Preface ix
About the authors xiii
Abbreviations xvii

High weighted questions 1
Medium weighted questions 54
Low weighted questions 73
Calculations questions 97
Case based discussion questions 110
High weighted answers 112
Medium weighted answers 144
Low weighted answers 158
Calculations answers 176
Case based discussion answers 190
Index 193

Preface

Welcome to *Pharmacy Foundation Assessment Questions 2*. We have compiled 400 questions to help support your revision and preparation for the foundation trainee examination. There is a mixture of both multiple choice (MCQ), extended matching (EMQ) and calculation questions.

The content has a balance of high-weighted, medium-weighted and low-weighted topics, which have been derived from the GPhC framework. It is important that you are familiar with this framework, here is a summary of some of the key points from the framework and how they relate to the examination.

There are two parts to the assessment:

Part 1 consists of 40 calculation questions and you have 2 hours to complete these using a calculator.
Part 2 of the assessment is 120 questions: 90 single best answer MCQ questions and 30 EMQ questions. You have 2.5 hours to complete these without the use of a calculator.

Reference sources are provided for both parts and examples are:
- BNF extracts
- Summary of product characteristics
- Diagrams and images
- Medication charts

Therapeutic areas
Questions in part 2 of the assessment that relate to clinical care are mapped to key therapeutic areas. However, an individual question may map to multiple therapeutic areas.

High weighted therapeutic areas:
- Cardiovascular system
- Nervous system
- Endocrine system
- Infection

Medium weighted therapeutic areas:
- Genito-urinary system
- Gastro-intestinal system
- Respiratory system
- Immune system and malignant disease
- Blood and nutrition

Low weighted therapeutic areas:
- Musculoskeletal system
- Eye Ear, nose, and oropharynx
- Skin
- Vaccines
- Anaesthesia

High Risk Drugs

Each assessment is likely to include at least one question on each of the following drugs or drug groups:
- antibiotics
- anticoagulants
- antihypertensives
- chemotherapy
- insulins
- antidiabetic drugs
- parenteral drugs
- drugs with a narrow therapeutic index
- non-steroidal anti-inflammatory drugs
- methotrexate
- opiates
- valproate.

Paediatrics

Around 20 per cent of questions in the assessment (both part 1 and part 2) will relate to paediatric patients.

Calculations

Each part 1 assessment is likely to include at least one calculation question involving each of the following:

- doses and dose regimens
- dosage and unit conversions
- estimations of kidney function
- displacement volumes and values
- concentrations (e.g. expressed as w/v, % or 1 in x)
- dilutions
- molecular weight
- using provided formulae
- infusion rates
- pharmacokinetics
- health economics
- quantities to supply

Some questions in part 1 will test underpinning pharmacy knowledge as well as calculations skill. Some questions in part 2 may also require calculation although these calculations will be possible without the use of a calculator.

Preparation advice

Here are some key tips about how best to approach preparing yourself for the assessment.

Prior to the assessment

1. Practice before the exam as often as you can (try to practice in timed online conditions if possible).
2. Use the GPhC framework and guidance to help support your revision.
3. Review GPhC feedback about previous sittings.
4. Revise high weighted topics initially then medium weighted and low weighted topics.
5. When revising, consider understanding theory and application in your role (rather than just memorising).
6. Ask for feedback from colleagues / peers / mentor if you are struggling to understand some topics.
7. Take regular breaks when completing revision in the few weeks prior to sitting the exam.
8. Learn how to use the Surpass system.
9. If you are concerned about your mental health or wellbeing – seek advice from your mentor / GP.

10. Ensure you have the items you need for the day (ID, approved calculator, water bottle etc).
11. Get a good night's sleep prior to the day of the exam.

During the assessment
1. Try to remain calm / relax before starting the paper.
2. Read each question thoroughly (twice if needed to consider or highlight the key components).
3. Consider the most appropriate option – there may be times where you are considering two options however consider the MOST appropriate in the given scenario.
4. Consider what your answer might be (prior to checking the options).
5. Consider key elements of the question which may help to deduce the answer e.g. temperature in infection.
6. Rule out options initially and try to narrow down to the most appropriate choices.
7. Map the answer to the patient / scenario.
8. Consider the theme when answering questions.
9. In some cases, with EMQ questions, the same answer can be used again.
10. Do not panic if you have difficulty with a question, move on and focus on the rest of the paper.
11. Try to ensure that you finish the paper in the allocated time.

Good luck for your exam and future career, wishing you all the best!

About the authors

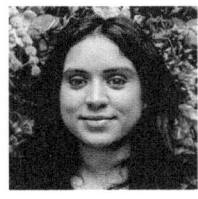

Sonia Kauser, MPharm, ClinDipHPharm, IP, ACP

Sonia Kauser is a portfolio pharmacist currently working for the University of Bradford as an Assistant Professor in medicine. Sonia enjoys teaching undergraduate and postgraduate students. Sonia is also a primary care educator for NHS England as well as an advanced prescribing pharmacist practitioner in primary care.

Sonia graduated from the University of Bradford and completed her pre-registration training at Bradford Teaching Hospitals NHS Foundation Trust. Sonia undertook training in various specialist clinical areas including cardiology, respiratory, psychiatry, general medicine, general surgery, vascular, orthopaedics, urology and paediatrics. Sonia undertook her postgraduate clinical diploma in hospital pharmacy during her time in hospital pharmacy.

Sonia then moved across to primary care where she started as a pharmacist in general practice. During this role she undertook chronic disease medication review clinics and undertaking weekly anticoagulation clinics. Sonia attained her independent prescribing and then moved onto studying the Advanced Clinical Practitioner diploma. She delivered weekly minor ailment clinics to support the GP surgery.

Sonia has worked for the University of Manchester as a senior lecturer in clinical pharmacy. Sonia was deputy lead for the pharmacist module and module lead for medicines management.

Sonia works with the Royal Pharmaceutical Society to deliver teaching sessions for foundation trainee pharmacists. Sonia is also starting a new role at the West Yorkshire ICB as a Senior Medicines Optimisation Pharmacist.

Sonia has previously worked in other sectors of pharmacy including community pharmacy, out of hours / urgent care and industry.

Sonia has written publications for the *International Journal of Pharmacy Practice*.

Sonia enjoys spending time with her three children and taking them for outdoor adventures.

Cam Anh Tran Phan, MPharm, PGDip Clinical Pharmacy Secondary Care, PGCert Psychiatric Therapeutics, PracCert Independent Prescribing, PCPEP ExemptCert, FHEA
Celia Feetam Award Winner 2019

Cam graduated from the University of Manchester and completed her pre-registration training at Bradford Teaching Hospitals NHS Foundation Trust. In her early career as a hospital pharmacist, Cam undertook training in various specialist clinical areas including psychiatry, general medicine, anticoagulation, cardiovascular, respiratory, general surgery, vascular, orthopaedic, urology and critical care. During this time, Cam successfully completed a PGDip in Clinical Pharmacy (Secondary Care) and a PGCert in Psychiatric Therapeutics. She was awarded the Celia Feetam Award in 2019 by the College of Mental Health Pharmacists for her outstanding performance on the PGCert in Psychiatric Therapeutics course at Aston University Birmingham.

Cam started her journey in academia as a guest lecturer in anticoagulation at the University of Bradford. With a strong passion for educating and developing future generation of pharmacists, Cam transferred into a permanent role as an Assistant Professor in Pharmacy Practice at the University. Within the MPharm programme, she has been the teaching lead for anticoagulation and cardiovascular diseases in Stage 3 and pharmaceutical calculations in Stage 4. In the last two years, Cam took on a pioneering role and co-led the development of the MPharm prescribing curriculum in alignment with the GPhC Initial Education and Training of Pharmacists (IETP) 2021. Cam's pedagogical interest lies in interprofessional education (IPE), and she has successfully developed various IPE activities within the Bradford MPharm programme in partnership with the Bradford College and the Leeds Medical School. Cam is recognised as a Fellow of the Higher Education Academy for her commitment to teaching and learning support in higher education.

Alongside her leadership and educational roles, Cam continues delivering patient-centred care as a pharmacist independent prescriber at the Porter Valley Primary Care Network in Sheffield. Maintaining her interest in anticoagulation and cardiovascular disease, Cam conducts a weekly clinic where she reviews and manages chronic patients in the community. Cam has also led a number of projects across general practice, enabling attainment of Quality and Outcomes Framework (QOF) and Network Contract Directed

Enhanced Service (DES) targets. She is currently developing a joint Foundation Training placement between primary care network and community pharmacy incorporating prescribing training in alignment with the GPhC IETP 2021.

Taking her research interest further, Cam is undertaking a PhD research project within the 'Supporting Safe Care in the Home' theme at the NIHR Yorkshire and Humber Patient Safety Research Collaboration

Cam has authored articles in the *Pharmaceutical Journal* and the *International Journal of Pharmacy Practice*. She has also been a presenter at the Royal Pharmaceutical Society (RPS) conference.

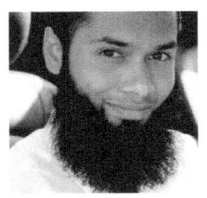

Habib Shah, MPharm, MRPharmS, Independent Prescriber

Habib Shah graduated from the University of Bradford in 2018 with a Master of Pharmacy. He completed his pre-registration training in a busy community pharmacy located within a medical centre, which provided him with early exposure to GP clinical setting. Upon qualifying, Habib took on the role of a GP Practice Pharmacist, where he was instrumental in implementing patient safety initiatives as well supporting the practice in meeting CQC standards.

In 2019, he joined Calderdale & Huddersfield NHS Foundation Trust as a clinical pharmacist, working across multiple specialties. During his time at the Trust, he also played a role in a unique pharmacy-led discharge service pilot that greatly enhanced both the speed and quality of patient discharges. Alongside his clinical work, Habib has been actively involved in education, contributing to the development of trainee pharmacists as the exam and calculations lead for Pharmacy Foundations. Through this role, he designs and delivers clinical training sessions to support future pharmacists at the University of Bradford.

In 2020, Habib started a role as a Primary Care Network (PCN) pharmacist, where he was promoted to senior pharmacist and co-lead of the trainee pharmacist programme in 2022. He also qualified as an independent prescriber in 2021, allowing him to provide greater care across both primary and secondary settings.

Habib's diverse experience across community pharmacy, general practice, and hospital environments made him a well-rounded portfolio pharmacist. His broad exposure in various healthcare settings positioned him as an ideal supervisor for trainee pharmacists in his PCN. He is also a member of the Yorkshire & Humber Trainee Pharmacist Advisory Group.

Committed to continuous professional development, Habib completed the Health Education England Primary Care Pharmacy Education Pathway and is currently training to become an anticoagulant specialist in primary care. His multifaceted expertise and dedication to improving patient care continue to drive his contributions to the profession.

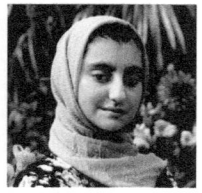

Misbah Noor Ansari, MPharm

Misbah Ansari graduated with a first-class honours from the University of Bradford School of Pharmacy in 2022. She completed the first six months of her foundation training with Woodroyd pharmacy, a busy community pharmacy in Bradford and the remaining six months in Harden pharmacy, a community pharmacy located in Harden village. She recently sat the registration exam in 2022, giving her a fresh understanding of the GPhC exam framework. Upon registration Misbah began to work for Lloyds pharmacy as a community pharmacist where she was as able to provide essential services. She is currently working as a locum pharmacist in West Yorkshire. Misbah enjoys learning new languages, reading and crocheting in her spare time.

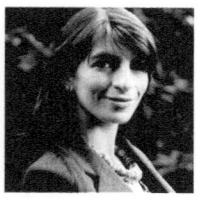

Sadia Qayyum, MPharm, PGCert Advanced Clinical Skills and Emergency Medicine, Independent Prescriber

Sadia boasts extensive experience across diverse sectors including retail, hospital, and general practice, holding management and consultancy roles. Currently, she serves as a lecturer in pharmacy practice at the University of Manchester, an independent prescriber in General Practice specialising in asthma, and a relief branch manager for Well. Her multifaceted background highlights her adeptness in evidence evaluation, decision-making, and communication. Committed to equity and diversity, she shapes policies and offers guidance in her various capacities. With a passion for professional development, Sadia engages in a wide range of speaking engagements, mentoring, and coaching healthcare professionals.

Sadia continues to work to highlight the unique and invaluable role pharmacists have in healthcare. Irrespective of pharmacists sector of work, she wishes to champion the notion that all pharmacists should aspire to lead the profession into the future.

Shaheen Razzaq, BScPharmacy (Hons), PGCert Advanced Clinical Skills and Emergency Medicine, Independent Prescriber (Contributor) Advanced Clinical Pharmacist Practitioner

Shaheen is currently working as the Clinical Lead of Pharmacists in general practice alongside her role as a practice pharmacist in primary care. Her pharmacy journey started in community pharmacy where she took up a management position early on in her career, she continued to want to progress in her role and therefore started the prescribing course which led her to the world of primary care. She has currently been working in primary care for 7 years and has explored the different areas including urgent care, general practice and out of hours services. She found herself orienting towards general practice and in committing to this journey is now a Clinical Lead overseeing and managing 7 Pharmacists whilst working alongside the clinical lead of other departments to ensure safety and efficiency in patient care. Her greatest goal is to ensure that patient safety is at the forefront of her whole practice and strives towards improving and finding ways to ensure she is constantly developing herself in this area.

Dillaver Rai is a primary care pharmacist who also helped contribute with question writing.

Abbreviations

ACBS	Advisory Committee on Borderline Substances
ACE	angiotensin-converting enzyme
ACEI	angiotensin-converting enzyme inhibitor
ACS	acute coronary syndrome
AF	atrial fibrillation
ALT DIE	alternate days
AV	arteriovenous
BD	twice daily
BMI	body mass index
BNF	*British National Formulary*
BNFC	*British National Formulary for Children*
BP	blood pressure
BPSA	British Pharmaceutical Students' Association
BSA	body surface area
BTS	British Thoracic Society
CCF	congestive/chronic cardiac failure
CD	controlled drug
CDC US	Centers for Disease Control and Prevention
CE	*conformité européenne*
CFC	chlorofluorocarbon
CHM	Commission on Human Medicines
CHMP	Committee for Medicinal Products for Human Use
CI	confidence interval or cumulative incidence
CKS	Clinical Knowledge Summaries
COX	cyclooxygenase
COPD	chronic obstructive pulmonary disease
CPD	continuing professional development
CPPE	Centre for Pharmacy Postgraduate Education
CrCl	creatinine clearance (mL/min)
CSM	Committee on Safety of Medicines
CYT	cytochrome
DigCl	digoxin clearance (L/h)
DMARD	disease-modifying antirheumatic drug
DNG	discount not given
DPF	Dental Practitioners' Formulary
DPI	dry-powder inhaler
EC	enteric-coated
ECG	electrocardiogram
EEA	European Economic Area
eGFR	estimated glomerular filtration rate

EHC	emergency hormonal contraception
F1	Foundation Year 1
FEV_1	forced expiratory volume in 1 second
GP	general practitioner
GP6D	glucose-6-phosphate dehydrogenase
GPhC	General Pharmaceutical Council
GSL	general sales list
GTN	glyceryl trinitrate
HbA1c	glycated haemoglobin
HDU	high dependency unit
HIV	human immunodeficiency virus
HR	heart rate
HRT	hormone replacement therapy
IBS	irritable bowel syndrome
IBW	ideal body weight
IDA	industrial denatured alcohol
IM	intramuscular
INR	international normalised ratio
IV	intravenous
IUD	intrauterine device
MAOI	monoamine oxidase inhibitor
MD	maximum single dose
MDD	maximum daily dose
MDI	metered-dose inhaler
MDU	to be used as directed
MEP	*Medicines, Ethics and Practice* guide
MHRA	Medicines and Healthcare products Regulatory Agency
MMR	measles, mumps and rubella
M/R	modified-release
MRSA	methicillin-resistant *Staphylococcus aureus*
MUPS	multiple-unit pellet system
MUR	Medicines Use Review
NHS	National Health Service
NICE	National Institute for Health and Care Excellence
NMS	New Medicines Service
NRLS	National Reporting and Learning System
NSAIDs	non-steroidal anti-inflammatory drugs
OC	oral contraceptive
OD	*omni die* (every day)
OM	*omni mane* (every morning)
ON	*omni nocte* (every night)
OP	original pack
OPAT	outpatient parenteral antibacterial therapy

ORT	oral rehydration therapy
OTC	over-the-counter
P	pharmacy
PAGB	Proprietary Association of Great Britain
PCT	primary care trust
PHE	Public Health England
PIL	patient information leaflet
pMDI	pressurised metered-dose inhaler
PMR	patient medical record
POM	prescription-only medicine
POM-V	prescription-only medicine – veterinarian
POM-VPS	prescription-only medicine – veterinarian, pharmacist, suitably qualified person
PPIs	proton pump inhibitors
PRN	when required
PSA	prostate-specific antigen
PSNC	Pharmaceutical Services Negotiating Committee
QDS	*quarter die sumendum* (to be taken four times daily)
RCT	randomised controlled trial
RE	right eye
RPS	Royal Pharmaceutical Society (formerly RPSGB)
SARSS	Suspected Adverse Reaction Surveillance Scheme
SCRIPT	Standard Computerised Revalidation Instrument for Prescribing and Therapeutics
SeCr	serum creatinine
SGLT2	sodium (Na+)/glucose co-transporter 2
SHO	senior house officer
SIGN	Scottish Intercollegiate Guidelines Network
SLS	selected list scheme
SOP	standard operating procedure
SPC	summary of product characteristics
SSRI	selective serotonin reuptake inhibitor
ST	an isoelectric line after the QRS complex of an ECG
STAT	immediately
TCA	tricyclic antidepressant
TDS	three times a day
TIA	transient ischaemic attack
TPN	total parenteral nutrition
TSDA	trade-specific denatured alcohol
U&E	urea and electrolyte count
UTI	urinary tract infection
VITAL	Virtual Interactive Teaching And Learning
WHO	World Health Organization

High weighted questions

Question 1 – 2 relate to the same patient:

1. A 53-year-old patient with a history of epilepsy has been newly started on an antiepileptic drug. Within four weeks of starting the new drug, the man presents at the emergency department with fever, a widespread skin rash, and tender lymphadenopathy. Point-of-care testings show elevated liver functions, agranulocytosis and thrombocytopenia. The working diagnosis is antiepileptic hypersensitivity syndrome. Which of the following medications is most likely the antiepileptic drug that the man has been started on?

    ☐ A Carbamazepine
    ☐ B Levetiracetam
    ☐ C Sodium valproate
    ☐ D Vigabatrin
    ☐ E Zonisamide

2. The relevant antiepileptic drug was withdrawn immediately. The patient is reviewed by a neurologist and an alternative antiepileptic drug is started. As recommended by the DVLA, how long should the patient withhold driving?

    ☐ A 1 month
    ☐ B 3 months
    ☐ C 6 months
    ☐ D 12 months
    ☐ E Until reviewed by a neurologist.

3. A 40-year-old man was admitted to the emergency department following a first tonic-clonic seizure. He has a history of asthma, depression and lower back pain. He is taking the following medications:
    - Soprobec (beclomethasone) 200micrograms/dose inhaler 1 puff twice a day

- Salbutamol 100micrograms/dose inhaler 2 puffs when required
- Mirtazapine 30mg at night
- Paracetamol 1g four times a day when required
- Tramadol 50mg-100mg four times a day when required
- St John's Wort (bought OTC)
- Co-amoxiclav 625mg TDS (currently on day 5 of a 7-day course for chest infection)

The patient drinks around 10 units of alcohol per week. There was no family history of collapses or seizures. On examination, the patient is back to normal. There is no abnormalities with his blood results, ECG and CT head scan performed in the emergency department. Which of the following medications is most likely to provoke his episode of seizure?

☐ A Beclomethasone
☐ B Co-amoxiclav
☐ C Mirtazapine
☐ D St John's Wort
☐ E Tramadol

4 A 68-year-old man, who has Parkinson's disease, is taking the following medications:
- Sinemet Plus (co-careldopa) 25/100mg TDS
- Sinemet CR (co-careldopa) 50/200mg at night
- Rotigotine 8mg/24 hours patches – one patch daily

The patient is an ex-smoker (15 cigarettes a day for 40 years, which is equivalent to 30-pack year). At the latest Parkinson's disease review, his wife reports that the patient has recently participated in risky day-trading investments. He has also spent a lot of time at the horse-races and made large purchases of unnecessary gadgets. These are new and unusual behaviours for him.

Which of the following is the most suitable recommended action?

☐ A Gradually reduce the dose of co-careldopa
☐ B Gradually reduce the dose of rotigotine

☐ C Immediately stop co-careldopa
☐ D Immediately stop rotigotine
☐ E Offer cognitive behavioural therapy

Antipsychotic drugs (questions 5 to 8)

For each of the following scenarios select the most appropriate course of action from the list. Each option may be used once, or more than once, or not at all.

☐ A Discontinue the antipsychotic treatment
☐ B Reduce the dose of the antipsychotic treatment
☐ C Start hyoscine hydrobromide up to 300microgram TDS
☐ D Start procyclidine hydrochloride 5mg TDS
☐ E Switch the antipsychotic treatment to amisulpride
☐ F Switch the antipsychotic treatment to aripiprazole
☐ G Switch the antipsychotic treatment to olanzapine
☐ H Switch the antipsychotic treatment to trifluoperazine

5   A 45-year-old man with schizoaffective disorder has recently been started on haloperidol 5mg three times a day. A week after starting haloperidol, the patient develops a high fever and muscle rigidity. He also appears confused and complains of profused sweating. His blood pressure is 155/88mmHg (from 123/79mmHg) and his pulse is 118bpm (from 79bpm).

6   A 59-year-old man, who has a background of bipolar disorder, obesity, type 2 diabetes mellitus and hypertension, is taking the following medications:
    - Amlodipine 10mg OD
    - Metformin 1g BD
    - Ozempic (Semaglutide) 1mg subcutaneous injection once weekly
    - Risperidone 4mg OD
    - Valproic acid 1.5g BD

He recently develops breast enlargement and galactorrhoea. A blood test is performed and shows hyperprolactinaemia.

7   A 28-year-old man with treatment-resistant schizophrenia who is taking clozapine 100mg daily. When attending the clozapine monitoring clinic, the patient reports troublesome drooling, which occurs both during the daytime and at night. The nighttime symptoms cause pillow wetting and disrupt his sleep.

8   A 76-year-old woman with schizophrenia has been on flupenthixol decanoate intramuscular injection 50mg every 4 weeks for 5 years. The schizophrenia is stable, and she has been in remission for the last 3 years. At her annual mental health review, the patient reported she has experienced episodes of involuntary facial movements including grimacing and tongue protrusion in the last month.

9   A 58-year-old woman had an ST-segment-elevation myocardial infarction two months ago. She has since made a good recovery but has experienced low mood, lack of enjoyment from her usual hobbies and a poor sleep pattern. The patient is diagnosed with post-MI depression and is offered cognitive behavioural therapy. She wishes to try medication as the symptoms are affecting her ability to work. Which of the following is the most appropriate antidepressant for this patient?

- ☐ A   Amitriptyline
- ☐ B   Lofepramine
- ☐ C   Mirtazapine
- ☐ D   Sertraline
- ☐ E   Venlafaxine

10 A 54-year-old woman with a background of hypertension, depression and substance misuse is on the following medications:
- Atorvastatin 20mg OD
- Ramipril capsule 10mg OD
- Citalopram tablet 40mg OD
- Methadone 1mg/ml oral solution 100ml OD
- Diazepam tablet 2mg TDS when required
- Ondansetron 4mg up to three times a day when required – started three days ago for nausea and vomitting.

The patient's routine ECG shows a QTc interval of 490ms. Which of the following drug regimens is likely to cause QTc prolongation in this patient?

- [ ] A Atorvastatin, ramipril, ondansetron
- [ ] B Citalopram, methadone and diazepam
- [ ] C Citalopram, methadone and ondansetron
- [ ] D Ramipril, citalopram and diazepam
- [ ] E Ramipril, methadone, and diazepam

Questions 11-13 relates to the same patient

11 A 47-year-old woman with bipolar affective disorder is on the following medications:
- Fluoxetine 40mg OD
- Lithium carbonate (Priadel) 400mg BD

The patient's ambulatory blood pressure monitoring shows an average 168/104 mmHg. What is the most appropriate antihypertensive drug for this patient?

- [ ] A Amlodipine
- [ ] B Bendroflumethiazide
- [ ] C Doxazosin
- [ ] D Losartan
- [ ] E Ramipril

12 The patient reports a cluster of symptoms including dry skin, cold hands and feet, weight gain, tiredness, and low mood. The symptoms have been present for the last couple of months. Which of the following is the most appropriate investigation for the patient's symptoms?

- [ ] A CT abdominal scan
- [ ] B Full blood count
- [ ] C Liver function test
- [ ] D Mini-mental state examination
- [ ] E Thyroid function test

13 Lithium is a narrow therapeutic index drug, with the target therapeutic concentration of 0.4 – 1mmol/L. The patient's lithium level is 0.25mmol/L. As such, her lithium carbonate (Priadel) dose is increased to 600mg BD. When should the next lithium level be taken?

☐ A One week after dose change, at 12 hours after dose
☐ B One week after dose change, at 6 hours after dose
☐ C Six hours after the first dose
☐ D Three days after dose change, at 12 hours after dose
☐ E Three days after dose change, at 6 hours after dose

Disease classification and risk scoring system (questions 14 to 17)

For each of the following scenarios select the most appropriate disease classification or risk scoring system. Each option may be used once, or more than once, or not at all.

☐ A CHA2DS2-VASc
☐ B GRACE
☐ C HAS-BLED
☐ D NEWS2
☐ E No disease classification or risk scoring system exists
☐ F NYHA
☐ G ORBIT
☐ H QRISK3

14 A 63-year-old woman is newly diagnosed with atrial fibrillation. You wish to assess her risk of major bleeding with anticoagulation using a scoring system recommended by the NICE guidance.

15 A 75-year-old man is admitted to the emergency department with chest pain and raised troponin. An ECG is performed and confirms non-ST elevation myocardial infarction. You wish to assess his 6-month mortality and risk of future cardiovascular events in order to determine the next step of management.

16 A 54-year-old man is newly diagnosed with heart failure. You wish to classify the extent of his heart failure based on severity of symptoms and limitation of physical activity.

17 A 58-year-old man with a previous history of angina and hypertension. You wish to assess his 10-year risk of future cardiovascular events.

Adverse Drug Reactions (questions 18 and 19)

Select from the list below the drug most likely to cause the adverse reaction for each scenario. Each option may be used once, more than once, or not at all.

- ☐ A Aspirin
- ☐ B Bisoprolol
- ☐ C Dapagliflozin
- ☐ D Isosorbide mononitrate
- ☐ E Metformin
- ☐ F Nicorandil
- ☐ G Pioglitazone
- ☐ H Semaglutide (Ozempic)

18 A 63-year-old man with a background of stable angina, has recently been started on an anti-anginal medication. The patient presents at the community pharmacy requesting an OTC treatment for mouth ulcers. Upon examination, the mouth ulcers appear as clusters of several large, deep, persistent ulcers with punched out edges.

19 A 75-year-old woman with a background of heart failure with reduced ejection fraction (left ventricle ejection fraction of 35%) and type II diabetes, has recently been started on a medication for both conditions. The patient is admitted to hospital with severe diarrhoea and vomiting following an episode of food poisoning. During the admission, this medication was withheld due to the risk of ketoacidosis.

Fragmin® (dalteparin sodium) injection (questions 20 to 21)

For each scenarios described below recommend a Fragmin® regimen. The patients have no known drug allergies or contraindications to Fragmin®. Select the most appropriate regimen from the options below. Each option may be used once, more than once or not at all.

You may use the SPC for Fragmin® (dalteparin sodium) 5000 IU solution for injection to help you: https://www.medicines.org.uk/emc/product/4247/smpc

☐ A Dalteparin sodium 2,500 units S/C OD
☐ B Dalteparin sodium 5,000 units S/C OD
☐ C Dalteparin sodium 12,500 units S/C OD
☐ D Dalteparin sodium 12,500 units S/C OD with anti-Xa level monitoring
☐ E Dalteparin sodium 15,000 units S/C OD
☐ F Dalteparin sodium 15,000 units S/C OD with anti-Xa level monitoring
☐ G Dalteparin sodium 18,000 units S/C OD
☐ H Dalteparin sodium 18,000 units S/C OD with anti-Xa level monitoring

20 A 65-year-old man with a background of prostate cancer was diagnosed with pulmonary embolism five weeks ago. He has been started on Fragmin (dalteparin sodium) subcutaneous injection since. The patient weights 85kg and has a CrCl of 71ml/min. Other urea and electrolytes, liver function tests and full blood counts are within normal range. His other medication includes primidone 250mg daily for essential tremor. The patient is to be continued on Fragmin® (dalteparin sodium) for the treatment of pulmonary embolism.

21 A 78-year-old woman who is admitted to hospital with confusion secondary to pyelonephritis. Whilst in hospital, she is expected to have reduced mobility relative to normal state. Her blood test shows a CrCl of 40ml/min. Other urea and electrolytes, liver function tests and full blood counts are within normal range. She weighs 41kg and is currently taking the following medications:
- Temocillin IV 2g BD for 48 hours then review
- Atorvastatin 20mg ON
- Amlodipine 5mg OM
- Paracetamol PO/IV 500mg QDS PRN

The patient is to be prescribed Fragmin® (dalteparin sodium) for venous thromboembolism prophylaxis.

22 A 67-year-old woman with a background of hypertension and type II diabetes, is taking the following medications:

- Atorvastatin 20mg OD
- Ramipril 5mg OD
- Omeprazole 20mg OD
- Metformin m/r 1g OD

The patient experienced a transient ischaemic attack (TIA) and requires secondary preventative measures. therapy. Her atorvastatin dose is increased to 40mg once a day. Her medical record shows a previous anaphylactic reaction with clopidogrel. Which of the following antiplatelet(s) should be started in place of clopidogrel?

- ☐ A Aspirin 75mg OD
- ☐ B Aspirin 75mg OD and dipyridamole m/r 200mg BD
- ☐ C Aspirin 75mg and ticagrelor 90mg BD
- ☐ D Dipyridamole M/R 200mg BD
- ☐ E Dipyridamole M/R 200mg BD and ticagrelor 90mg BD

23 A 47-year-old woman, who was diagnosed with breast cancer, underwent a course of chemotherapy treatment. Six months after completion of chemotherapy, the patient develops a cluster of symptoms including oedema in her feet and ankles, shortness of breath on physical exertion, orthopnoea and paroxysmal nocturnal dyspnoea. An echocardiogram is performed which shows a left ventricle ejection fraction (LVEF) of 45% - a reduction by 30% from her baseline. Which of the following chemotherapy agents has most likely caused the patient's presentation?

- ☐ A 5-Fluorouracil
- ☐ B Bleomycin
- ☐ C Cyclophosphamide
- ☐ D Doxorubicin
- ☐ E Gemcitabine

Questions 24 and 25 relate to the same patient:

24 A 70-year-old man with a background of prosthetic valve replacement (30 years ago), hypertension, angina and atrial fibrillation, is admitted from home to hospital with shortness of breath, generalised muscular aches, fever, night sweats and a petechial rash. On history taking, it is discovered that he had a tooth extraction two weeks ago.

The patient is diagnosed with infective endocarditis and is started on antibiotics. His blood pressure on admission is 94/56 mmHg. His heart rate is 56bpm. He weighs 80kg. He has no known drug allergies and his current medication is listed below:
- Ramipril capsule 5mg OD
- Rivaroxaban tablet 15mg OD (with meal)
- Verapamil (Half Securon SR) tablet 240mg BD

Which of the following drugs is it most important to withhold temporarily in view of his current blood pressure and heart rate?

☐ A Atorvastatin
☐ B Paracetamol
☐ C Ramipril
☐ D Rivaroxaban
☐ E Verapamil (Half Securon SR)

25 For the treatment of endocarditis, the patient was commenced on flucloxacillin IV 2g four times a day, rifampicin 600mg PO twice a day and gentamicin 500mg IV stat. Which of the following drugs must be changed upon the introduction of antibiotic therapy?

☐ A Atorvastatin
☐ B Paracetamol
☐ C Ramipril
☐ D Rivaroxaban
☐ E Verapamil (Half Securon SR)

26 Mrs K has been prescribed simvastatin tablets to control her cholesterol levels. She also takes amlodipine 5mg tablets for hypertension. What is the maximum daily dose of simvastatin that this patient can take?

☐ A 10mg
☐ B 20mg
☐ C 40mg
☐ D 80mg
☐ E None of the above

27 Mrs J, age 56, has just been discharged from hospital after suffering from a myocardial infarction (NSTEMI). The patient has been started on a atorvastatin. Which other medications would you expect the patient to have been started on as secondary prevention of cardiovascular events?

☐ A Aspirin with clopidogrel
☐ B Atenolol
☐ C Ramipril
☐ D All of the above
☐ E None of the above

Questions 28 and 29 relate to the same patient:

28 Miss H, aged 34, is 27 weeks pregnant. She has developed hypertension during her pregnancy. Which of the following medications is the most appropriate to treat her hypertension?

☐ A Amlodipine
☐ B Labetalol
☐ C Losartan
☐ D Propranolol
☐ E Ramipiril

29 A few months pass by and Miss H has now given birth. She has chosen to breastfeed her baby. Which of the following medications should she be switched to?

☐ A Amlodipine
☐ B Bendroflumethiazide
☐ C Candersartan
☐ D Enalapril
☐ E Methyldopa

30 Mrs CG (age 42 years) takes a calcium channel blocker for her atrial fibrillation. She is attending her cardiology review to consider uptitrating her medication. Which of the following calcium channel blockers should not be used alongside beta-blockers?

☐ A Amlodipine
☐ B Diltiazem
☐ C Felodipine
☐ D Nifedipine
☐ E Verapamil

31 You are a primary care pharmacist working in the lipid clinic. You are due to review Mrs GT today and are considering the initiation of a statin due to raised cholesterol levels (6.2 mmol/l). You have various statin tablets you can choose from. Which one of the following statins is classed as medium intensity?

☐ A Atorvastatin 80mg
☐ B Fluvastatin 80mg
☐ C Pravastatin 40mg
☐ D Rosuvastatin 40mg
☐ E Simvastatin 80mg

32 You are a foundation pharmacist and are preparing a powerpoint presentation for junior doctors in secondary care. You are teaching them about digoxin. Which of the following statements regarding digoxin is incorrect?

☐ A Digoxin is indicated for atrial fibrillation
☐ B Electrolytes and renal function must be monitored
☐ C For plasma-drug concentration, blood should be taken at least 4 hrs after a dose
☐ D The dose of digoxin should be reduced by half if used alongside amiodarone
☐ E Yellow – green vision is a sign of toxicity

Questions 33 - 38 describe scenarios for specific patients.

Select the most appropriate drug regimen from the options below. Each option may be used once, more than once or not at all.

☐ A Azithromycin
☐ B Cefalexin

- [ ] C Clarithromycin
- [ ] D Co-Amoxiclav
- [ ] E Doxycycline
- [ ] F Flucloxacillin
- [ ] G Gentamicin
- [ ] H Metronidazole

33 A 45-year-old male with diabetes develops a foot infection

34 A 25-year-old female with suspected diverticulitis

35 A 6-year-old child with a penicillin allergy develops otitis media

36 A 23-year-old female with bacterial vaginosis

37 A 44-year-old female who has been bitten by her dog

38 A 30-year-old male with non-severe hospital acquired pneumonia

39 You are a microbiology pharmacist and are currently reviewing a patient who is prescribed long term antibiotics. Which of the following antibiotics requires skin protection?

- [ ] A Cefalexin
- [ ] B Clarithromycin
- [ ] C Doxycycline
- [ ] D Flucloxacillin
- [ ] E Metronidazole

40 Miss LT (age 4 years) is admitted onto the A and E ward due to query meningitis. Which of the following cephalosporins is used for treating infections of the central nervous system such as meningitis?

- [ ] A Cefalexin
- [ ] B Ceftaroline
- [ ] C Ceftazidime
- [ ] D Ceftriaxone
- [ ] E Cerfuroxime

41 You are a junior pharmacist working on the aseptics unit. You have been asked to prepare gentamicin for a patient who is currently on the vascular ward. Using the SPC provided, which of following regarding gentamicin is incorrect?

- [ ] A Caution is advised when driving due to possible undesired effects of vertigo
- [ ] B Gentamicin can be diluted with 0.9% sodium chloride or 10% glucose solution
- [ ] C Gentamicin is eliminated unchanged in microbiologically active form Ceftriaxone
- [ ] D It is contraindicated in myasthenia gravis
- [ ] E Vomiting is a very common side effect

42 You are a community pharmacist, and a patient presents with a dental prescription due to an infected abscess. Upon reviewing the prescription, you note you may need to counsel the patient on alcohol use with this medication. Which of the following antibiotics can cause a dilsufuram-like reaction if taken with alcohol?

- [ ] A Ciprofloxacin
- [ ] B Clarithromycin
- [ ] C Co-amoxiclav
- [ ] D Metronidazole
- [ ] E Rifampicin

43 You are a junior pharmacist working in hospital. You work on the cardiology ward and during a ward round, you notice a patient complaining of muscle pains. You speak to the on-call doctor and a suggestion is made of rhabdomyolysis due to recently started medication. Which medication could be causing this?

- [ ] A Fluticasone
- [ ] B Paracetamol
- [ ] C Prednisolone
- [ ] D Simvastatin
- [ ] E Tramadol

44 Mrs. YZ, aged 54, has experienced a recent myocardial infarction (MI) and is currently grappling with depression as a result. Her GP has recommended the use of an SSRI as per NICE guidance to manage her low mood. Among the available SSRIs, which one is considered the safest for an individual who has recently had a MI?

☐ A Citalopram
☐ B Escitalopram
☐ C Fluoxetine
☐ D Paroxetine
☐ E Sertraline

45 Mr AB (age 62 years) is admitted into the hospital following muscle fatigue, weakness, arrhythmias, nausea. His potassium levels are 6.4 mmol/L and is diagnosed with hyperkalaemia. Which medication needs to be withheld due to hyperkalaemia?

☐ A Folic acid
☐ B Ibuprofen
☐ C Ramipril
☐ D Sertraline
☐ E Terbutaline

46 You are junior pharmacist working on the nephrology ward. You are discussing the interactions of foods and medicines with the team. Which of the following medicine is most likely to have an interaction with grapefruit juice?

☐ A Atenolol
☐ B Ciclosporin
☐ C Naproxen
☐ D Rivaroxaban
☐ E Rosuvastatin

47 Mrs PG (age 58 years) has been discharged from hospital following a transient ischaemic attack. She notes discomfort related to muscle pain after her discharge. Which of the following medicines is likely to be the cause?

☐ A Aspirin
☐ B Atenolol
☐ C Bezafibrate
☐ D Clopidogrel
☐ E Omeprazole

48 A 67-year-old female patient with a medical history of: asthma, type II diabetes, hypertension and ischaemic heart disease has been hospitalised due to an exacerbation of her asthma. She has no documented drug allergies. You are reviewing her inpatient prescription chart. You note the following medication:
- Aspirin, tinzaparin, Seretide® inhaler, salbutamol inhaler, lisinopril, isosorbide dinitrate.

The patient is complaining of flushing and headaches. Which medicine may be causing this?

☐ A Aspirin
☐ B Isosorbide monitrate
☐ C Lisinopril
☐ D Seretide® inhaler
☐ E Tinzaparin

49 You are a junior pharmacist working on the medical admissions unit. You have been asked to suggest a beta-blocker for a patient who typically experiences cold extremities. Which would be most appropriate?
Literature available – BNF, Beta blocker summary - https://bnf.nice.org.uk/treatment-summaries/beta-adrenoceptor-blocking-drugs/

☐ A Atenolol
☐ B Bisoprolol
☐ C Labetalol
☐ D Pindolol
☐ E Propranolol

50 You are a working on the cardiology ward as a hospital pharmacist. The junior doctor is seeking guidance concerning a patient's medication history following an ECG. The doctor is inquiring whether any of the medications the patient is currently taking cause QT prolongation. Which of the following medication could be causing this?

☐ A Citalopram
☐ B Furosemide
☐ C Loratadine
☐ D Paracetamol
☐ E None of the above

51 You are a community pharmacist working at your regular pharmacy. A 30-year-old female patient began taking 200mg of lithium once daily for bipolar disorder under her GP's care two months ago. She is experiencing nausea and severe diarrhoea. She has recently had a prescription for flucloxacillin 500mg four times a day for cellulitis, which you initially believe is the cause for these gastro-intestinal effects. You question further and discover that she has taken an unintentional double dose of lithium tablets yesterday. What is the most appropriate advice for this patient?

☐ A Consider an alternative antibiotic to abate the gastrointestinal effects
☐ B Continue all medicines as prescribed
☐ C Halve the dose of lithium today to counteract the double dose from yesterday
☐ D Recommend loperamide to stabilise the loose motions
☐ E Stop lithium and to seek urgent medical attention

52 You are a primary care pharmacist undertaking a pain clinic and Mrs VN (37 years) attends today to discuss her analgesia options. Her past medical history is bipolar disorder and she takes lithium for management. Which of the following could cause risk when taken with lithium for pain relief?

☐ A Diclofenac
☐ B Nefopam
☐ C Oxycodone
☐ D Paracetamol
☐ E Tramadol

53 Mr. DR, a 56-year-old man weighing 60kg, has been admitted to the hospital due to an epileptic seizure. He has a medical history of myocardial infarction, mild depression and epilepsy. His blood parameters are otherwise normal. Mr Dr would like to reduce his medication because he is being considered for anti-epileptic medication. Which is the safest to prescribe?

☐ A Aspirin
☐ B Bisoprolol
☐ C Isosorbide mononitrate
☐ D Losartan
☐ E Sertraline

54 You are a Clinical Commissioning group pharmacist. You are helping the local formulary team write the pain management guidelines. Which of the listed medications can counteract the pain-relieving effects of other opioids?

☐ A Buprenorphine
☐ B Oxycodone
☐ C Naproxen
☐ D Paracetamol
☐ E Tramadol

55 You are a primary care pharmacist and the nurse practitioner is requesting your advice regarding antibiotics for her patient. Her patient is a 28-year-old male with a history of tendon damage. He has no known drug allergies. Which of the following drugs should she avoid using with this patient?

☐ A Amoxicillin
☐ B Ciprofloxacin
☐ C Doxycycline
☐ D Flucloxacillin
☐ E Oxytetracycline

56 You are working in a minor ailments clinic and your patient Miss SG (28 years) is complaining of headaches. You ask the appropriate questions,

and she informs you her pain has been present on the left side of her head (near temporals) and she has experienced some nausea. She has not been sick. Miss G is on no other medication nor suffers from any other conditions. She reports no other symptoms. Which of the following is your initial working diagnosis?

☐ A Aneurysm
☐ B Migraine
☐ C Rebound headache
☐ D Temporal arteritis
☐ E Tension headache

57 Following the MHRA alert in November 2017, antiepileptic drugs should be prescribed according to brand specific products, depending on which category the drug belongs to. Which epileptic medicine would you dispense as the same brand?

☐ A Brivaracetam
☐ B Carbamazepine
☐ C Clobazam
☐ D Ethosuximide
☐ E Levetiracetam

58 You are a primary care pharmacist reviewing a patient. You notice they have been prescribed a long-term proton pump inhibitor (pantoprazole). They recently complained of loose stools, nausea and stomach cramps. They were subsequently seen by their GP and a stool sample revealed they had C. difficile infection. Which of the following would be the *immediate* cause of action to take?

☐ A Prescribe ciprofloxacin
☐ B Prescribe clindamycin
☐ C Prescribe fidaxomicin
☐ D Stop the pantoprazole
☐ E Switch the pantoprazole to a less potent proton pump inhibitor

59 A 14-year-old patient is prescribed benzoyl peroxide for his acne vulgaris. Which of the following is appropriate advice regarding the use of his gel?

☐ A Apply appropriate sunscreen if there is sun exposure
☐ B Apply QDS
☐ C Apply QDS and PRN
☐ D Can only apply if taking oral antibiotic medication for acne alongside treatment
☐ E Continue to apply if severe irritation occurs

60 Mrs. GH (72 years) visits the pharmacy and reports symptoms of dysuria, fever, and flank pain. She is not taking any medication and does not suffer from any long term conditions. She has not tried anything over the counter. What is the most appropriate course of action?

☐ A Supply clotrimazole 1% cream
☐ B Supply cystitis relief sachets
☐ C Supply fluconazole capsules
☐ D Supply paracetamol and cystitis relief sachets
☐ E Refer the patient to the GP

61 You are working as a pharmacist and are counselling a patient who has been diagnosed with tuberculosis (TB). They understand that they have been prescribed isoniazid for TB. You also notice they have been prescribed pyridoxine. They think the pyridoxine has been prescribed in error. You explain that it has been prescribed to mitigate:

☐ A Glucose fluctuations
☐ B Nausea
☐ C Neuropathy
☐ D Sunlight related skin rashes
☐ E Tremors

62 Miss KJ, a 45-year-old patient, is admitted into hospital due to infection symptoms (fever, malaise, rigours). Which of the following blood tests can help deduce if the symptoms are related to an infection?

- A B12
- B Colecalciferol
- C CRP
- D Folate
- E Serum drug levels

63 You are working closely with the senior pharmacist at the HIV outpatients clinic. The team has decided to initiate a protease inhibitor for a newly diagnosed patient. Which of the following medication is recommended?

- A Isoniazid
- B Methotrexate
- C Mycophenolate
- D Pyridoxine
- E Ritonavir

64 You are a rotational hospital pharmacist and currently working on the renal ward. Patient AM, a 68-year-old male, has been noted to have a decline in renal function. His eGFR is now 28 mL/minute/1.73 m². Which medicine would you consider stopping?

- A Amlodipine
- B Linagliptin
- C Metformin
- D Nifedipine
- E Tramadol

Questions 65 and 66 are related to the same patient.

65 You are a hospital pharmacist helping to review patients. On today's ward round Mrs BZ, a 56-year-old female patient, complains of tiredness, paraesthesia, mouth ulcers, and a sore and red tongue. Her past medical history is type II diabetes, hypertension and hypercholesterolaemia. Which medicine would you review initially?

- A Ibuprofen
- B linagliptin

- [ ] C Metformin
- [ ] D Paracetamol
- [ ] E Simvastatin

66 What monitoring would you suggest is the most appropriate in this case?

- [ ] A Colecalciferol
- [ ] B Folate levels
- [ ] C Liver function tests
- [ ] D Vitamin B12
- [ ] E Zinc

You are a primary care clinical pharmacist conducting a diabetes clinic. The questions 67 to 71 are related to various patients who present to the clinic.

67 Today you are speaking to Mrs CF (age 57 years). She has been initiated on metformin 500mg once daily (two weeks ago). She recently titrated up to 500mg twice daily. Her recent eGFR is 40 mL/minute/1.73 m2. On presentation, she is complaining of nausea, abdominal pain, a fast heart rate and rapid breathing. Upon examination you note a low blood pressure reading. What would be the most appropriate next step?

- [ ] A Continue on the same dose until the symptoms subside
- [ ] B Decrease the dose of metformin to 500mg once daily
- [ ] C Increase the dose of metformin to TDS
- [ ] D Stop the metformin and seek urgent advice from the GP
- [ ] E Switch the metformin to modified release to reduce side effects

68 Miss LT (age 43 years) is a type 2 diabetic patient. She presents to the diabetes clinic for a routine review. She is complaining of rapid weight gain. Which medicine is most likely to have caused this?

- [ ] A Empagliflozin
- [ ] B Gliclazide
- [ ] C Linagliptin
- [ ] D Metformin
- [ ] E Semaglutide

69 Mr EB is 78-year-old male suffering with type II diabetes, heart failure, glaucoma, and erectile dysfunction. His current BP is 118/78mmHg and he is having an increasing trend in the HbA1c levels. His current medication is metformin 1g BD. You want to add another medication to lower the HbA1c. Mr EB agrees to the step-wise management. Which medicine should be avoided?

☐ A Dapagliflozin
☐ B Gliclazide
☐ C Linagliptin
☐ D Liraglutide
☐ E Pioglitazone

70 Mr. TT, a 67-year-old male suffering from type II diabetes has attended the diabetes clinic. You are discussing complications with diabetes, and he mentions that he has been getting more frequent thrush-like symptoms. Which of the following medication is the most likely cause?

☐ A Acarbose
☐ B Empagliflozin
☐ C Gliclazide
☐ D Linagliptin
☐ E Metformin

71 Mr GH is a 75-year-old male with type II diabetes, asthma and hypertension. He has recently started a new medicine for optimal diabetic control. You are concerned with the symptoms he is describing (nausea, vomiting, abdominal pain, dark urine, and itchy skin.) Which medication do you consider stopping immediately?

☐ A Amlodipine
☐ B Fluticasone
☐ C Metformin
☐ D Pioglitazone
☐ E Salbutamol

72 While working on the orthopaedic ward, you conduct a medication review on a patient who has presented with an atypical humerus fracture.

This patient has been taking his medication consistently for 10 years. You are scrutinising his medication and advise the doctors which might be the probable cause of this fracture?

☐ A Aspirin
☐ B Bisoprolol
☐ C Gliclazide
☐ D Felodipine
☐ E Risedronate

73 You are a community pharmacist. A patient has been prescribed bromocriptine for acromegaly. They are unsure how long they will be taking the medication for, and the prescriber has asked you to counsel the patient. Which counselling point is relevant to the patient?

☐ A Do not take the medication after 6pm
☐ B Do not take with paracetamol
☐ C Report any rashes to your dentist
☐ D This medication can cause low mood
☐ E You may experience hypotension when initially prescribed this, your blood pressure should be monitored

74 Patients should be advised to promptly inform healthcare providers of any indications of bone marrow suppression (such as flu-like symptoms) associated with various medications listed in the British National Formulary (BNF). Which of the following drugs is associated with bone marrow suppression?

☐ A Mebendazole
☐ B Melatonin
☐ C Methocarbamol
☐ D Methotrexate
☐ E Methyldopa

75 Miss. FG presents with to A&E with a swollen moon-shaped face, stretch marks on her abdomen and facial acne. Which medication is most likely to be contributing to these symptoms?

- A Bisoprolol
- B Cyanocobalamin
- C Levothyroxine
- D Methylprednisolone
- E Paracetamol

76 Miss KS (age 24 years) is diagnosed with hypothyroidism. This is based on her recent thyroid stimulating hormone (TSH) and T4 levels. Which of the following symptoms could indicate hypothyroidism in a patient?

- A Being sensitive to cold and gaining weight
- B Feeling hot and losing weight
- C Feeling more elated/happier than usual
- D Irregular heartbeat
- E Loose stools

Questions 77, 78 and 79 are related to the same patient.

77 Mr AS, a 61 year old male patient of Afro-Carribean descent, has recently been discharged from hospital with nil medication changes. His recent bloods were in range. His blood pressure was raised. He is currently prescribed:
- Amlodipine 5mg - Take ONE daily due to stage 1 hypertension.

The practice nurse checks his blood pressure today and it is now 151/92. Home Blood Pressure Monitoring is requested. Which of the following readings would be within target of Stage 1 hypertension?

- A <120/80
- B <130/80
- C <150/80
- D <140/94
- E <150/90

78 His average home BP reading is 149/91. What is the most appropriate next step to add for the patient?

- A Bisoprolol 5mg tablet OD
- B Furosemide 20mg tablet OD

- [ ] C Ramipril 1.25mg tablet OD
- [ ] D Ramipril 10mg tablet OD
- [ ] E Spironolactone 25mg tablet OD

79 Mr AS has been commenced on the most appropriate medication. You have requested follow up in two weeks. What are you monitoring?

- [ ] A Blood pressure
- [ ] B Blood pressure and pulse check
- [ ] C Blood Pressure, U&E and LFT
- [ ] D Blood Pressure, U&E and side effects
- [ ] E HbA1c, U&E, LFT, FBC

80 Mrs SA a 29-year-old caucasian woman has recently been initiated on sodium valproate 200mg tablet - ONE to be taken TWICE a day by the neurologist, the indication states for migraine prophylaxis. The neurologist has asked you to take over prescribing of this medication. Which of the following statements is TRUE with regards to further management of this patient?

- [ ] A Sodium valproate is licensed for use in migraine prophylaxis
- [ ] B The GP should consider prescribing propranolol 80mg m/r capsules instead of sodium valproate
- [ ] C The GP should ensure the patient is signed up for the Pregnancy Prevention Programme, explaining the risks associated with the medication
- [ ] D The GP should take over prescribing of the sodium valproate because the neurologist has reviewed the patient and deems it appropriate
- [ ] E The patient is 29 and of child bearing age, the GP should prescribe the sodium valproate but should review the patient and discuss the teratogenic risks of sodium valproate in pregnancy

81 Mr. PL a 72-year-old Caucasian male is undergoing a clinical medication review. He is currently prescribed:
- Ramipril 10mg OD
- Citalopram 40mg OD
- Paracetamol 500mg - 1-2QDS PRN

Which of the statements below is FALSE with regards to the medication?

- ☐ A Citalopram is also available as Cipramil® 40mg/ml drops and 4 oral drops (8mg) is equivalent in therapeutic effect to 10mg tablet
- ☐ B GP should consider stopping the prescribing of paracetamol as it can be bought over the counter, since the patient is using it when required
- ☐ C GP should consider switching citalopram 40mg to escitalopram 20mg OD in patients over 65
- ☐ D Patient is on ramipril so patients blood pressure and U&E should be monitored annually
- ☐ E When reviewing medication, pharmacist should ensure that patient is not taking any other agents over the counter that contain paracetamol

82 You are a primary care clinical pharmacist. Mr OL a 59 year old Pakistani male, has requested an acute prescription for zopiclone 7.5mg tablets ONE to be taken at night. He is currently not taking any medication. You check his records and note that he has been issued 4 week's worth a year ago. What is the most appropriate way to manage this request?

- ☐ A Advise GP to issue zopiclone 3.75mg OD and titrate up to zopiclone 7.5mg OD if ineffective at the lower dose
- ☐ B Advise GP to prescribe promethazine instead as it is a sedating antihistamine and therefore less addictive than Z-Drugs
- ☐ C Book in with GP for review - it has been a year since patient last had this medication issued and will need to be reviewed by GP to see if medication is appropriate
- ☐ D Do not issue the medication as the patient has already taken up to 4 week's worth of medication and therefore can no longer request further issue
- ☐ E Issue the zopiclone since the patient has had it before and therefore is aware of how to use it. It is clear the patient is not misusing the drug as last issue was a year ago

83 Mrs JK a 49-year-old Caucasian woman has recently started a new medication. A week later she presents with a fever, some bruising on her

arms and legs and widespread mouth ulcers in her mouth. On examination you note that this is side effect of her most recent medication that needs to be stopped immediately. What is the medication that would have most likely contributed to these symptoms?

☐ A   Carbamazepine
☐ B   Carbimazole
☐ C   Chlorphenamine
☐ D   Clobazam
☐ E   Clonazepam

84 Mr. HM, a 47-year-old Caucasian male, has been experiencing severe migraines. His GP has recently prescribed him prophylactic treatment to prevent the migraines. He has been booked in with you for a medication review at the primary care clinic. He complains of recently experiencing nightmares. What prophylactic migraine medication is likely to have caused this?

☐ A   Amitriptyline
☐ B   Bisoprolol
☐ C   Propranolol
☐ D   Timolol
☐ E   Topiramate

85 Mr IP, a 38-year-old Afro-Carribean male, has been experiencing severe pain. He is reviewed by his GP who diagnosed it as neuropathic pain. He is given a prescription for:
• Amitriptyline 10mg tablet - Take ONE daily.

He asks you what the common side effects of the drug are. What is the most appropriate response?

☐ A   Diarrhoea and Vomiting
☐ B   Dry mouth, constipation and urinary retention
☐ C   Hair loss
☐ D   Hyperactivity
☐ E   Hypersalivation

86 Mr PT, an 89-year-old Caucasian male, is experiencing nausea and vomiting. He is a palliative care patient. The doctor has asked you what dose of metoclopramide he should prescribe? What is the most appropriate dose for this patient?
The BNF monograph is available here - https://bnf.nice.org.uk/drugs/metoclopramide-hydrochloride/#indications-and-dose

- A 10mg STAT
- B 10mg TDS
- C 10mg every 6 hours
- D 30-100mg/24 hours
- E Up to 500mcg/kg daily in 3 divided doses

87 Mr JK a 35-year-old Caucasian man has started on olanzapine 5mg tablets - Take ONE daily. Prior to starting the medication, he was requested to be booked in for baseline bloods and management. Which bloods and management should have been requested?

- A BP check, U&E/eGFR, HbA1c, serum lipids, LFT
- B HbA1c and full blood count
- C HbA1c, BP check and height
- D Serum lipids and weight
- E U&E/eGFR and height

88 Mr AF a 67 year old Caucasian man has presented to their GP complaining of muscular back pain. The GP issued a prescription for diclofenac m/r 75mg tablet - Take ONE twice a day. His medical conditions are:
- atrial fibrillation
- migraines

Which of the following statements is FALSE?
The BNF monograph for diclofenac is available here – https://bnf.nice.org.uk/drugs/diclofenac/

- A An increased risk of heart attack and stroke with diclofenac is well recognised particularly with long-term use of high doses and in patients who are already at high risk

- B Hair colour changes with topical use of diclofenac
- C Long term use of diclofenac is associated with reduced female fertility, which is reversible on stopping treatment
- D The correct dose of diclofenac for muscular back pain is 75mg/mr tablet - Take ONE three times a day
- E Topical application of large amounts of diclofenac can result in systemic effects

89 You are a community pharmacist. Mrs SL, a 39-year-old Asian female, has pregabalin for peripheral neuropathic pain on her repeat medication. A medication request has come through to you for the following:
- Pregabalin 150mg capsule - Take ONE twice a day

What is incorrect with regards to this prescription?

- A Pregabalin is not indicated for peripheral neuropathic pain
- B Pregabalin is only available as tablets
- C The dose of pregabalin is incorrect for peripheral neuropathic pain
- D The quantity of pregabalin is incorrect
- E There is nothing incorrect with this prescription

90 Mr PN, an 81-year-old caucasian male, has been prescribed Madopar® CR capsules 100/25 m/r capsules TWO three times a day for Parkinsons. He has recently been struggling with his swallowing and the GP has requested that you change his medication to dispersible tablets. When switching from modified release levodopa to dispersible co-beneldopa, approximately how much should the dose be reduced by?

- A 5%
- B 10%
- C 25%
- D 30%
- E The dose does not need to be reduced

For questions 91 to 95 select the most likely medication. Each option may be used once, more than once or not at all.

- ☐ A Empagliflozin
- ☐ B Gliclazide
- ☐ C Glucotabs
- ☐ D Humulin M3
- ☐ E Linagliptin
- ☐ F Metformin
- ☐ G Novorapid insulin vials
- ☐ H Pioglitazone

91 Mrs GK a 72-year-old Caucasian woman has recently had her bloods checked, everything returned as normal apart from her blood glucose levels. Her recent HbA1c was 75mmol/mol. During her appointment with her GP she was prescribed a medication. The GP has advised her of the risk of hypoglycaemia associated with this drug especially when taking other glucose-lowering drugs. Given this information what drug was this patient most likely prescribed?

92 Miss WL a 24-year-old Caucasian woman has recently been diagnosed with polycystic ovary syndrome (PCOS). She has been prescribed a medication. When she gets home she reads the patient information leaflet and it states it is a glucose-lowering drug. She rings the pharmacy confused as to why she has been prescribed this medication and says she thinks it may be a mistake. You assure her it isn't a mistake and that this drug is used in the treatment of PCOS. What drug is this most likely to be?

93 This drug inhibits dipeptidylpeptidase-4 to increase insulin secretion and lower glucagon secretion.

94 Mrs LS, a 91-year-old Caucasian woman experienced a fall and was nil-by-mouth for a few days. Her diabetes medication was not omitted. She then went into diabetic ketoacidosis. Which drug most likely caused this?

95 Which drug should be stopped in the elderly when the eGFR is less than 30ml/minute/1.73m2 due to the risk of lactic acidosis?

96 Mrs WQ, a 45-year-old Asian woman, is currently prescribed:
   - Paracetamol 500mg tablets - Take ONE or TWO four times a day when required
   - Naproxen 500mg tablets - Take ONE twice a day after food when required
   - Lansoprazole 15mg capsules - Take ONE daily when taking naproxen
   - Carbimazole 20mg - Take ONE daily

   She presents to the community pharmacy complaining of a sore throat and a more than usual pain in her muscles. What is the most appropriate management plan for this patient?

   ☐ A Advise patient to attend A&E immediately
   ☐ B Advise patient to book in for routine GP review and in the interim to take honey, lemon and ginger mixture to help with sore throat
   ☐ C Advise patient to continue taking naproxen and paracetamol which should help with her sore throat and to consider increasing fluid intake and rest
   ☐ D Advise patient to see her GP immediately for review and blood test
   ☐ E Offer patient benzydamine sore throat spray and advise to increase fluid intake and rest

97 Miss TR, a 34-year-old Caucasian woman, has seen the GP today and has been started on levothyroxine 25mcg tablets - Take ONE daily, she was asymptomatic and opportunely her recent blood tests have revealed that she is hypothyroid. The doctor has requested that you arrange monitoring for this patient, what is the most appropriate monitoring plan for this patient?

   ☐ A Measure FT4 every 3 months and then 6 monthly thereafter
   ☐ B Measure TSH levels monthly until stable and then 6 monthly thereafter
   ☐ C Measure TSH levels every 3 months until a stable level has been achieved then yearly thereafter
   ☐ D Measure TSH levels annually
   ☐ E Measure both TSH and FT4 levels every three months and then 6 monthly thereafter

98 Mrs LK, a 65-year-old woman, has been prescribed a medication for her bones. The GP has advised her that she needs to take this medication on an empty stomach and stand or sit upright for at least 30 minutes after taking this medication. What is this drug most likely to be?

☐ A Adcal® D3 tablets
☐ B Alendronic acid tablets
☐ C Glucosamine tablets
☐ D Naproxen tablets
☐ E Paracetamol tablets

99 Mrs SW a 24-year-old Asian woman presents to the pharmacy with redness in her left eye, it waters regularly and is a little painful, she explains in the morning she wakes up and it is crusty and sticky; she uses a flannel and cool boiled water to wipe away the residue. She has had this for two days. She is not on any other medication. What is the most appropriate treatment for this patient?

☐ A Advise patient to continue with what she is currently doing as it is self-limiting and should resolve soon. If it doesn't within 5 days, she should return
☐ B Chloramphenicol 0.5% eye drops - one drop every 2 hours for 2 days then reduce to 4 hourly
☐ C Chloramphenicol 1% eye ointment - apply 3-4 times a day
☐ D Fusidic Acid 1% eye gel - use twice a day
☐ E See GP immediately

100 A 5-year-old Caucasian child presents to the pharmacy with his mother. She shows you his mouth, there are reddish sores with orange, honey-coloured crusty patches on it. She is concerned with regards to this. Based on the description what is it most likely to be?

☐ A Chicken pox
☐ B Contact dermatitis
☐ C Herpes simplex
☐ D Impetigo
☐ E Scabies

101 Mrs KT, a 78-year-old Caucasian woman, has requested a home visit from the GP. She complains of pain when urinating and feeling the need to go but being able to urinate. On examination the GP notices that she has a fever of 38.5 degrees, rigors and she has been vomiting. The GP carries out an abdominal examination and finds that she has costovertebral angle tenderness. He prescribes cefalexin 500mg TDS for 10 days. Which of the following is a correct statement regarding cefalexin?

☐ A Anaphylaxis is a common side effect
☐ B Avoid in urinary tract prophylaxis infections
☐ C Avoid in pregnant patients
☐ D Cross sensitivity does not occur with penicillins
☐ E False positive urinary glucose tests have been reported

102 Mr LP an 85-year-old Caucasian man is struggling with his breathing and finds that he is wheezing. He has COPD. The GP examines him and discovers that it is an acute exacerbation of COPD. What statement below is FALSE with regards to COPD and its treatment?

☐ A About up to 50% of cases are viral, 30-50% are bacterial and the remaining tests are undetermined. Antibiotics are not indicated in the absence of purulent/micropurulent sputum especially if not associated with increased dyspnoea.
☐ B Long term oral corticosteroid is usually recommended at the lowest dose possible. Patients should be monitored for osteoporosis.
☐ C NICE (2019) recommends to send a sputum sample for culture and susceptibility testing and then offer an antibiotic.
☐ D The main risk factor for development and exacerbations of COPD is tobacco smoking. Other risk factors include environmental pollution and occupational exposures.
☐ E Together with the patient, action plans should be created for those at risk of exacerbations. In patients who have had an exacerbation within the last year, a short course of antibacterials and oral corticosteroids should be kept at home.

103 Miss SS, a 63-year-old Asian woman has recently been travelling to the Far East. She presents with an ache in her stomach, feelings of nausea

associated with a loss of appetite and bloating. The GP carries out some tests and from the findings issues her a prescription for:
- Lansoprazole 30mg BD for 7 days
- Amoxicillin 1g for 7 days
- Clarithromycin 500mg BD for 7 days

Based on the prescription what is the most likely diagnosis?

☐ A Crohns Disease
☐ B Gastroenteritis
☐ C H-Pylori
☐ D Gastroenteritis
☐ E Travellers diarrhoea

104 On receiving the prescription at the Pharmacy you ask Miss SS if she is allergic to penicillin. She says yes immediately and proceeds to tell you she got really sick the last time it was issued. You contact the GP to inform him. He changes the prescription. In patients with this diagnosis, what is the most appropriate treatment for patients with a penicillin allergy?

☐ A Lansoprazole 30mg BD for 7 days
Cefalexin 500mg BD for 7 days
Clarithromycin 500mg BD for 7 days
☐ B Lansoprazole 30mg BD for 7 days
Doxycycline 100mg STAT then OD for 7 days
Clarithromycin 500mg BD for 7 days H-Pylori
☐ C Lansoprazole 30mg BD for 7 days
Metronidazole 400mg BD for 7 days
Clarithromycin 500mg BD for 7 days
☐ D Lansoprazole 30mg BD for 7 days
Tetracyline 500mg QDS for 7 days
Clarithromycin 500mg BD for 7 days
☐ E Lansoprazole 30mg BD for 14 days
Clarithromycin 500mg BD for 14 days

105 Miss SS is on a medication that the doctor has requested the patient stop until the treatment is over due to its interaction with Clarithromycin 500mg BD. Which drug is this most likely to be?

☐ A Allopurinol
☐ B Fluoxetine
☐ C Gabapentin
☐ D Naproxen
☐ E Simvastatin

For question 106 to 110 select the most likely medication. Each option may be used once, more than once or not at all.

☐ A Desogestrel
☐ B Estraderm Mx patch
☐ C Estradiol pessary
☐ D Ethinylestradiol 30mcg/Levonorgestrel 50mcg
☐ E Etonogestrel implant
☐ F Intra-uterine contraceptive device
☐ G Levonorgestrel
☐ H Norethisterone

106 Miss LS, a 28-year-old caucasian woman has attended an appointment at the GP practice. She is going on her honeymoon in two weeks to the Maldives and is requesting a medication to postpone menstruation. Which medication is used to postpone menstruation?

107 Miss AK, a 25-year-old Asian woman has requested a progesterone only contraceptive pill to be taken daily. Which is the most appropriate medication for this request?

108 Miss AW, a 23-year-old Caucasian woman comes in to your pharmacy requesting the morning after pill. Which medication is used for the morning after pill?

109 Mrs JP, a 38-year-old Caucasian woman attends the GP practice with extreme pain in her abdomen which seems to be swollen, she is vomiting and seems to have a fever., she gave birth a year ago and is currently breastfeeding The GP sends her to the hospital. At the hospital, after some tests and an ultrasound they have diagnosed her with uterine perforation. Which of the medication is most likely to have caused this?

110 Miss IP, a 29-year-old Caucasian woman, wants to commence on a contraceptive pill. She requests that she doesn't 'have the pill that gives you a clot'. On further questioning you find out that her friend developed venous thromboembolism from taking the contraceptive pill. Which of the medication is she most likely referring to?

111 Mr HL, a 68 year old Caucasian man, has been prescribed finasteride 5mg tablets - Take ONE daily for benign prostatic hyperplasia. A lower dose of this drug can also be used for what other condition?

☐ A Androgenetic alopecia in men
☐ B Erectile dysfunction
☐ C Priapism
☐ D Pulmonary Hypertension in men
☐ E Varioceles

112 Mrs YR, a 59-year-old Caucasian woman, presents to the GP complaining of vaginal dryness and pain during sexual intercourse. She is requesting something to alleviate the symptoms. She is on no other medication. What is the most appropriate treatment for this patient?

☐ A Clotrimazole 500mg pessaries
☐ B Clotrimazole 2% cream
☐ C Fluconazole 50mg capsules
☐ D Metronidazole 400mg tablets
☐ E Replens® MD moisturiser

113 Mr. HB, a 48-year-old Caucasian man, presents to the GP with erectile dysfunction. He is requesting a drug that will allow him to engage in spontaneous sexual activity rather than scheduled. Which drug should this patient be commenced on?

☐ A Avanafil 100mg
☐ B Finasteride 5mg
☐ C Sildenafil 50mg
☐ D Tadalafil 5mg
☐ E Vardenafil 10mg

114 Mrs WA, a 34-year-old Caucasian woman, presents to the GP complaining of a white discharge that smells 'fishy'. She is currently pregnant. On examination the GP diagnoses this as bacterial vaginosis. What is the most appropriate treatment option for this patient?

☐ A Clotrimazole 10% vaginal cream 5g single dose
☐ B Fluconazole 150mg STAT
☐ C Metronidazole vaginal gel 0.5% nightly for 5 nights
☐ D Metronidazole 400mg QDS for 7 days
☐ E Metronidazole 4g STAT

115 Ms PA, 35 years old, presented to the GP complaining of itching and irritation in the vaginal area associated with a cottage-cheese-like discharge. On examination the GP states she has vulvovaginal candidasis. What statement is FALSE with regards to vulvovaginal candidasis?

☐ A Acute vulvovaginal candidasis is treated with an antifungal drug such as fluconazole or with intravaginal imdazole pessary or cream inserted high in to the vagina
☐ B If a pregnant woman develops vulvovaginal candidasis she will need a shorter duration of treatment to ensure safety of the foetus
☐ C Intravaginal imidazole drugs are effective against candida in short courses of 1 - 14 days according to the preparation used
☐ D Recurrence of vulvovaginal candidasis is particularly likely if there are predisposing factors such as recent (up to 3 months before) antibacterial therapy, and poorly controlled diabetes
☐ E Vulvovaginal candidasis, also known as genital thrush, is symptomatic inflammation of the vagina and or vulva caused by a superficial fungal infection - *candida albicans*

116 Mr HP (62 years) has a raised QRISK score (20%) and a history of raised lipid levels. Which of the following medicines is most commonly prescribed for the primary prevention of cardiovascular events in patients with hyperlipidemia?

☐ A Aspirin
☐ B Enalapril

- C Furosemide
- D Metoprolol
- E Simvastatin

117 A 55-year-old male with a history of hypertension is prescribed amlodipine for stage 1 hypertension. He receives his medication for the first time, which of the following is a common side effect associated with this medication?

- A Bradycardia
- B Dry cough
- C Hyperkalemia
- D Peripheral oedema
- E Weight loss

118 Mrs TF (48 years) has a history of heart failure. Which of the following statements is correct about the use of ACE inhibitors in heart failure?

- A They are contraindicated in patients with diabetes
- B They are less effective than angiotensin 11 receptor blockers (ARBs) in reducing mortality
- C They can cause a persistent dry cough as a side effect
- D They require routine drug level monitoring
- E They should always be combined with beta-blockers

119 A patient presents with chest pain at A&E, upon review he is diagnosed with a STEMI. Which medication is typically given as part of the initial management?

- A Aspirin
- B Atorvastatin
- C Digoxin
- D Furosemide
- E Ramipril

120 Which of the following medicines is used as a first-line treatment for chronic stable angina. It can improve the patients' symptoms by reducing the heart rate and myocardial oxygen consumption?

- [ ] A Bisoprolol
- [ ] B Diltiazem
- [ ] C Furosemide
- [ ] D Glyceryl trinitrate
- [ ] E Nifedipine

121 Miss PF (14 years) is diagnosed with asthma following symptom review and a peak flow diary. Which of the following is a long-acting beta2 agonist (LABA) used in the management of asthma?

- [ ] A Budesonide
- [ ] B Ipratropium
- [ ] C Montelukast
- [ ] D Salbutamol
- [ ] E Salmeterol

122 Miss GS (28 years old) with asthma is prescribed Clenil® inhaler. Which of the following is a common side effect of inhaled corticosteroids?

- [ ] A Diarrhoea
- [ ] B Hypertension
- [ ] C Hypokalemia
- [ ] D Oral candidiasis
- [ ] E Weight gain

123 You are running an asthma clinic with the primary care centre. Master JH (age 7 years) presents with mum. Mum is unsure which medication is the preventor, and which is the reliever. Which of the following is usually recommended as first-line treatment for the relief of acute asthma symptoms?

- [ ] A Salmeterol
- [ ] B Montelukast
- [ ] C Salbutamol
- [ ] D Prednisolone
- [ ] E Theophylline

124 Mr MW (62 years) is diagnosed with COPD due to a 25-year history of smoking. He is prescribed ipratropium for as-and-when use. What is the mode of action of his new medication?

☐ A Beta2 receptor agonist
☐ B Blocks reabsorption of serotonin
☐ C Glucocorticoid receptor agonist
☐ D Leukotriene receptor antagonist
☐ E Muscarinic receptor antagonist

125 Mr LT (23 years) has been managing his asthma with his reliver use following exercise. However recently he has noted an increase in symptoms which also affect him at night. The GP reviews him and decides to commence preventative medication. Which of the following would be the most likely choice of medication?

☐ A Clenil® inhaler
☐ B Ipratropium inhaler
☐ C Montelukast
☐ D Prednisolone tablets
☐ E Salbutamol inhaler

126 Mr AP (53 years) is diagnosed with type II diabetes. His BMI is 35 kg/m2. Which of the following would be the most appropriate to start for Mr AP?

☐ A Gliclazide
☐ B Insulin glargine
☐ C Linagliptin
☐ D Metformin
☐ E Pioglitazone

Question 127 to 129 relate to the same patient.

127 Miss KC (24 years) presents to the GP clinic with feeling of tiredness. The GP requests blood test monitoring and following her TSH results, she is diagnosed with sub-clinical hypothyroidism. Which of the following medications is most likely to be prescribed to manage her condition?

- ☐ A Colecalciferol
- ☐ B Ferrous sulphate
- ☐ C Folic acid
- ☐ D Levothyroxine
- ☐ E Propylthiouracil

128 Which of the following is a side effect of her new medication?

- ☐ A Arrythmias
- ☐ B Confusion
- ☐ C Constipation
- ☐ D Hyperkalaemia
- ☐ E Weight gain

129 Which of the following is related to over-replacement of her new medication?

- ☐ A Bradycardia
- ☐ B Hyperglycemia
- ☐ C Hypotension
- ☐ D Osteoporosis
- ☐ E Weight gain

130 Mr LT (61 years old) is prescribed hydrocortisone long term for his Addison's disease. You receive the prescription request in your community pharmacy. Which of the following is the most appropriate counselling for Mr LT?

- ☐ A Always carry a steroid treatment card
- ☐ B Continue on the same dose during illness
- ☐ C It is best to take this dose at night
- ☐ D Reduce the dose during illness
- ☐ E Stop if you develop any side effects

131 Mr LG (age 33 years) is prescribed carbimazole to manage his hyperthyroidism. Which of the following adverse reactions would need an immediate referral to secondary care?

- A Agranulocytosis
- B Diarrhoea
- C Headache
- D Hyperkalaemia
- E Hypoglycaemia

132 Mrs FG (56 years) has a history of type II diabetes. She presents to the primary care clinic with a raised average home BP (148/95). A urine sample also suggests albuminuria. You decide to commence treatment for this patient. Which drug would you commence this patient on?

- A Amlodipine
- B Bisoprolol
- C Indapamide
- D Nifedipine
- E Ramipril

133 Mr VP (age 72 years) has undergone surgery and has had a mitral valve replacement. He has a history of atrial fibrillation, and it is recommended he is prescribed warfarin long term. Which of the following monitoring would be undertaken to ensure he is receiving the correct dose?

- A ECG
- B Full blood count
- C INR levels
- D Liver function tests
- E Urea and electrolytes

134 Mrs LF (67 years) has been diagnosed with an NSTEMI. Which of the following medicines would most likely be prescribed for the patient to take long term (upon discharge)?

- A Aspirin, amlodipine, bisoprolol, digoxin, warfarin
- B Aspirin, clopidogrel, furosemide, atorvastatin, ramipril
- C Aspirin, clopidogrel, ramipril, bisoprolol, atorvastatin
- D Rivaroxaban, clopidogrel, atorvastatin, furosemide, spironolactone
- E Rivaroxaban, warfarin, furosemide, atorvastatin, digoxin

135 Mr LG (62 years) is prescribed a new medication to help manage his heart failure due to reduced ejection fraction. You review his blood results today and they are as follows:
- Potassium – 6mmol/L
- Sodium – 137mmol/L
- Urea – 3mmol/L

Which of the following may have contributed to this reading?

☐ A Apixaban
☐ B Bisoprolol
☐ C Bisoprolol
☐ D Furosemide
☐ E Spironolactone

136 Miss LG (23 years) is currently 16 weeks pregnant. She presents to your primary care clinic reporting urinary discomfort. Upon reviewing, you diagnose her with an uncomplicated urinary tract infection. She has no known allergies. Which of the following would be the most appropriate medication to issue?

☐ A Ciprofloxacin
☐ B Clarithromycin
☐ C Doxycycline
☐ D Lymecycline
☐ E Nitrofurantoin

Questions 137 to 139 relate to the same patient.

137 Mrs PS (59 years) attends your primary care clinic, complaining of feeling unwell and a chesty cough. Upon reviewing, you note she is pyrexial, breathless and bronchial breath sounds. She has no known drug allergies. You diagnose her with community-acquired pneumonia. Which scoring system helped you deduce the diagnosis?

☐ A Centor
☐ B Chads2Vasc2 score

- C CRB-65
- D HAS-BLED score
- E QRISK

138 What is the most appropriate management plan?

- A Advise self-care and offer amoxicillin
- B Advise self-care remedies and paracetamol
- C Prescribe ciprofloxacin
- D Prescribe clarithromycin
- E Prescribe doxycycline

139 What is a common side effect of your chosen first line treatment?

- A Altered liver function tests
- B Confusion
- C Diarrhoea
- D Nephrotoxicity
- E Tendonitis

Questions 140 and 141 relate to the same patient.

140 Miss CO (33 years) has a history of type 1 diabetes. She has a history of repeated oral candidiasis. Which of the following antifungal medications is commonly used as treatment?

- A Itraconazole
- B Ketoconazole
- C Metronidazole
- D Miconazole
- E Terbinafine

141 If there was treatment failure or the infection was extensive, which of the following would be an appropriate alternative?

- A Fluconazole
- B Itraconazole

- ☐ C Ketoconazole
- ☐ D Miconazole
- ☐ E Terbinafine

Questions 142 and 143 relate to the same patient.

142 Miss KC (22 years) presents to the minor ailments clinic at the primary care clinic. She complains of foul-smelling discharge over the last 2 weeks. There is nil itching in the genital area. Upon examination there is no soreness. She is not pregnant, had nil medical history. Based on the examinations, what is the most likely diagnosis?

- ☐ A Allergy
- ☐ B Atrophic vaginitis
- ☐ C Bacterial vaginosis
- ☐ D Chlamydia
- ☐ E Vaginal candidiasis

143 Given this diagnosis which of the following would be appropriate first-line therapy?

- ☐ A Clotrimazole
- ☐ B Fluconazole
- ☐ C Metronidazole
- ☐ D Nitrofurantoin
- ☐ E Trimethoprim

144 Mr GT (age 58 years) is admitted onto the respiratory ward with an infective exacerbation of COPD. 3 days later he reports loose stools and feeling thirsty. Upon clinician review, he is diagnosed with *clostridioides difficile*. Which of the following would be an appropriate choice of first line treatment?

- ☐ A Amoxicillin
- ☐ B Doxycycline
- ☐ C Itraconazole
- ☐ D Metronidazole
- ☐ E Vancomycin

145 Mr JW (age 23 years) presents to the primary care clinic as he is struggling to control his worries. He also experiencing restless and irritability. With his university undergraduate exams approaching, he is struggling to sleep or to concentrate. He is diagnosed with generalised anxiety disorder. Which of the following would be the most appropriate medication treatment?

- ☐ A Diazepam
- ☐ B Lorazepam
- ☐ C Methylphenidate
- ☐ D Sertraline
- ☐ E Venlafaxine

146 Mr AJ (age 27 years) is diagnosed with a manic psychotic episode (first presentation). His past medical history includes asthma and psoriasis. The mental health team initiate him on olanzapine at 2.5mg OD. Which of the following is a common side effect of this drug?

- ☐ A Diarrhoea
- ☐ B Hypercalcaemia
- ☐ C Hyperglycaemia
- ☐ D Hyperkalaemia
- ☐ E Hypertension

147 Miss SW (age 34 years) is diagnosed with major depressive disorder. She has had previous treatment failure with a SSRI therefore it is decided to commence a SNRI for symptom management. Which of the following is an appropriate choice of medication?

- ☐ A Amitriptyline
- ☐ B Lofepramine
- ☐ C Mirtazapine
- ☐ D Paroxetine
- ☐ E Venlafaxine

148 Mrs PW (age 82 years) is a palliative care patient. You are the community pharmacist and have been asked to review her medication. Which of the following adverse effects is commonly associated with one of her medicines (amitriptyline)?

☐ A Dry mouth
☐ B Hypocalcaemia
☐ C Hypokalaemia
☐ D Hypomagnaseia
☐ E Weight gain

149 Mis ST (28 years) is struggling with insomnia due to a family bereavement. The GP has decided to initiate zolpidem to manage her insominia. Which of the following is a CORRECT statement regarding zolpidem?

☐ A Take 10mg OD for up to 2 weeks
☐ B Take 10mg OD for up to 4 weeks
☐ C Take 10mg OD for up to 8 weeks
☐ D Take 10mg OD for up to 12 weeks
☐ E Take 10mg OD for up to 16 weeks

150 Miss LP (25 years) presents to the community pharmacy complaining of a migraine. Her past medical history is migraine with aura since age 13. She has no known drug allergies. Her migraine has lasted 24 hours. Which of the following is a correct statement regarding the OTC sale of sumatriptan?

☐ A Sumatriptan can be supplied to anyone between the ages of 18-75 years
☐ B Sumatriptan can be supplied to patients with a history of epilepsy
☐ C Sumatriptan can be used as preventative treatment as well as during an acute attack for patients aged 18 years and older
☐ D Take one tablet at the onset of a migraine, if there is no symptom relief then another tablet can be taken after 2 hours
☐ E The maximum dose is 4 tablets in a 24 hour period

Questions 151 to 155 relate to the same patient.

151 Miss FR (42 years) is initiated on lithium following a mental health review with a secondary care consultant. Which of the following diagnosis would be an appropriate indication?

☐ A Treatment of acute schizophrenia
☐ B Treatment of bipolar disorder

- C Treatment of dementia
- D Treatment of generalised anxiety disorder
- E Treatment of mild depression

152 Which of the following is recommended as routine monitoring for lithium?

- A Lithium drug levels, eGFR, thyroid levels
- B Lithium drug levels, liver function tests, eGFR
- C Liver function tests, eGFR, thyroid levels
- D Liver function tests, full blood count, eGFR
- E None of the above

153 What is a common side effect of long-term lithium use?

- A Hypertension
- B Lethargy
- C Memory impairment
- D Sleep disturbances
- E Weight loss

154 What are the routine recommended serum-lithium concentration levels?

- A 0.2 – 1 mmol/L
- B 0.4 – 1mmol/L
- C 0.4 – 1.2mmol/L
- D 0.6 – 1mmol/L
- E 0.6 – 1.2mmol / L

155 6 months later, Miss FR is diagnosed with hypertension. Her GP recommends changes to her lifestyle and provides dietary advice. Which of the following is a CORRECT statement regarding dietary advice?

- A Maintain adequate fluid intake, avoid dietary changes which reduce or increase iron intake
- B Maintain adequate fluid intake, avoid dietary changes which reduce or increase magnesium intake
- C Maintain adequate fluid intake, avoid dietary changes which reduce or increase potassium intake

☐ D Maintain adequate fluid intake, avoid dietary changes which reduce or increase sodium intake
☐ E Maintain adequate fluid intake, avoid dietary changes which reduce or increase zinc intake

Antidepressant medication (questions 156 to 160).

For each of the following scenarios select the most appropriate option from the list. Each option may be used once, or more than once, or not at all.

☐ A Amitriptyline
☐ B Fluoxetine
☐ C Lithium
☐ D Mirtazapine
☐ E Paroxetine
☐ F Sertraline
☐ G Trazodone
☐ H Venlafaxine

156 A 36-year-old patient requires an anti-depressant medication. He has previously trialled an SSRI. The desired effect would be to manage his depression and sleep at night. Which would be the most appropriate next step to trial?

157 An SSRI type of medication with a long half-life and the preferred treatment choice in depression in children.

158 An SSRI type of medication with a short half-life and associated with a higher risk of withdrawal symptoms.

159 An antidepressant usually chosen first line due to safety reasons for patients with a history of cardiovascular disease.

160 A presynaptic alpha2-adrenoreceptor antagonist which increases central noradrenergic and serotonergic neurotransmission.

Antibiotic medication (questions 161 to 165).

For each of the following scenarios select the most appropriate option from the list. Each option may be used once, or more than once, or not at all.

- ☐ A Amoxicillin
- ☐ B Azithromycin
- ☐ C Ciprofloxacin
- ☐ D Doxycycline
- ☐ E Flucloxacillin
- ☐ F Gentamicin
- ☐ G Lymecycline
- ☐ H Trimethoprim

161 A patient is diagnosed with cellulitis in primary care and this is recommended as first line treatment.

162 Cholestatic jaundice and hepatitis can occur up to two months after treatment.

163 There is a risk of ototoxicity and nephrotoxicity when prescribing this medication.

164 There is a risk of inducing convulsions when prescribing this medication.

165 There is risk of tendon damage when prescribing this medication.

Cardiovascular (questions 166 to 170).

For each of the following scenarios select the most appropriate option from the list. Each option may be used once, or more than once, or not at all.

- ☐ A Amiodarone
- ☐ B Amlodipine
- ☐ C Clopidogrel
- ☐ D Digoxin
- ☐ E Diltiazem

☐ F Furosemide
☐ G Spironolactone
☐ H Warfarin

166 A patient is admitted onto a stroke ward following a transient ischaemic attack. This medication is prescribed long term on discharge.

167 This drug can be used for atrial fibrillation and atrial flutter, drug levels not recommended unless toxicity suspected and ideally check drug levels at least 6 hours post dose.

168 A chest x-ray is required prior to initiating treatment with this drug, it is recommended to monitor liver function tests and thyroid function tests during treatment.

169 A patient has chronic heart failure and this drug is prescribed to try to reduce fluid overload.

170 Counsel patient on serious adverse reactions affecting the eyes, heart, lung, liver, thyroid gland, skin, and peripheral nervous system which can persist for a month or after treatment discontinuation.

Diabetes (questions 171 to 175).

For each of the following scenarios select the most appropriate option from the list. Each option may be used once, or more than once, or not at all.

☐ A Canagliflozin
☐ B Dulaglutide
☐ C Glimepiride
☐ D Insulin glargine
☐ E Metformin
☐ F Ozempic
☐ G Pioglitazone
☐ H Sitagliptin

171 An overweight patient is newly diagnosed with type II diabetes mellitus; they are going to be initiated on a first-line oral agent that works by reducing hepatic glucose production. Which medicine is the most appropriate choice?

172 A GLP-1 receptor agonist which is to be prescribed once weekly for self-administration by subcutaneous injection in the thigh, abdomen, or upper arm, rotating the injection sites between doses.

173 A patient requires a second drug for the management of their type II diabetes. This drug would be avoided due to the patient's history of heart failure.

174 The MHRA has warned regarding a serious risk of this medicine being sold as a 'fake medicine'.

175 Prior to initiating treatment with this drug, you need to check whether the patient may be at increased risk of diabetic ketoacidosis and if they have a low carbohydrate diet.

Medium weighted questions

176 Women of childbearing potential should avoid handling crushed or broken tablets of which drug?

☐ A Finasteride
☐ B Sildenafil
☐ C Tadalafil
☐ D Terazosin
☐ E Vardenafil

177 Miss F has recently been prescribed Microgynon® 30 tablets. Which of the following would not be a reason to stop the COC immediately? The SPC is available here: https://www.medicines.org.uk/emc/product/1130/smpc

☐ A First time occurrence of migraines
☐ B Onset of nausea
☐ C Pain and swelling of the leg
☐ D Severe upper abdominal pain
☐ E Sudden disturbances of vision

178 Which of the following counselling points is CORRECT regarding MR tamsulosin tablets?

☐ A Avoid indigestion remedies 2 hours before or after taking this medicine
☐ B Do not crush or chew
☐ C Protect your skin from sunlight
☐ D Take 30 to 60 minutes before food
☐ E Take with a full glass of water

179 Within how many hours of the unprotected sexual intercourse (UPSI) can a copper inter-uterine device be fitted?

☐ A 24 hours
☐ B 36 hours
☐ C 72 hours
☐ D 120 hours
☐ E 144 hours

180 How often should clotrimazole 2% cream be applied for vaginal thrush?

☐ A Once daily
☐ B One or two times a day
☐ C Twice daily
☐ D Two or three times a day
☐ E Four times a day

Gastrointestinal System (questions 181 to 188).
For each of the following scenarios select the most appropriate option from the list. Each option may be used once, or more than once, or not at all.

☐ A Co-danthramer
☐ B Docusate Sodium
☐ C Isphaghula Husk
☐ D Lactulose
☐ E Linaclotide
☐ F Macrogol
☐ G Methylnaltrexone bromide
☐ H Senna

181 This drug increases intestinal motility and often causes abdominal cramps but is not restricted to the use of terminally ill patients.

182 This laxative decreases surface tension.

183 This laxative consists of inert polymers of ethylene glycol which sequester fluid in the large bowel.

184 This drug is licensed for the treatment of moderate to severe irritable bowel syndrome associated with constipation.

185 This laxative should be avoided in patients with opioid induced constipation.

186 Which laxative can be used in the treatment of hepatic encephalopathy?

187 This drug is only licensed to be used to treat constipation in terminally ill patients.

188 This laxative can be supplied over the counter to a pregnant patient who is suffering with constipation.

189 Which of the following is NOT a characteristic of Crohn's disease?

☐ A   Abdominal pain
☐ B   Diarrhoea
☐ C   Diffuse mucosal inflammation
☐ D   Fever
☐ E   Rectal bleeding

Inhaler Active Ingredients (questions 190 to 195).
For each of the following inhalers select the most appropriate active ingredients from the list. Each option may be used once, or more than once, or not at all.

☐ A   Beclomethasone dipropionate with formoterol fumarate and glycopyrronium bromide
☐ B   Beclometasone with formoterol
☐ C   Fluticasone with formoterol
☐ D   Fluticasone with salmeterol
☐ E   Fluticasone with umeclidinium bromide and vilanterol
☐ F   Glycopyrronium bromide
☐ G   Mometasone furoate with gylcopyrronium bromide and indacaterol
☐ H   Salbutamol

190 Ventolin Evohaler®

191 Seebri Breezhaler®

192 Trimbow®

193 Flutiform®

194 Trelegy Ellipta®

195 Seretide Accuhaler®

196 Miss NF visits the pharmacy to collect her child's prescription for a spacer device. Which of the following pieces of advice is correct?

☐ A Spacer devices are compatible with all inhalers
☐ B Spacer devices increase the velocity of the aerosol
☐ C Spacer devices should be replaced every 3 months
☐ D Spacer devices remove the need for coordination
☐ E The spacer device should be cleaned once a week

197 Master J, aged 17, suffers from asthma. He is currently using salbutamol as reliever therapy and a low dose ICS for maintenance therapy. Despite these two therapies, his asthma remains uncontrolled. In line with NICE guidelines, what would be the most suitable add on therapy?

☐ A Formoterol
☐ B Increasing the dose of ICS
☐ C MART (maintenance and reliever therapy)
☐ D Montelukast
☐ E Salmeterol

198 Which of the following antihistamines is the most sedating?

☐ A Alimemazine
☐ B Ceterizine
☐ C Chlorphenamine
☐ D Cyclizine
☐ E Loratadine

199 Which of the following is the correct dose of adrenaline for a 8-year-old child in the emergency treatment of anaphylaxis?

☐ A   100 – 150 micrograms
☐ B   150 micrograms
☐ C   250 micrograms
☐ D   300 micrograms
☐ E   500 micrograms

200 Mr A, aged 30, has just been prescribed Clenil Modulite® 200mcg/dose inhaler. Which of the following counselling points are the most appropriate?

☐ A   Breathe steadily and deeply
☐ B   Rinsing the mouth immediately after each dose can prevent thrush
☐ C   The inhaler should be cleaned once a week
☐ D   All of the above
☐ E   None of the above

201 What is the correct dose of folic acid for a lady wishing to become pregnant and with a high risk of neural tube defects?

☐ A   400mcg daily, before conception and continue until week 12
☐ B   5mg daily, before conception and until term
☐ C   5mg daily, before conception until week 12 of pregnancy
☐ D   5mg daily until term
☐ E   5mg once weekly

202 Tingling in the lips, fingers/feet and tongue are all signs of which electrolyte abnormality?

☐ A   Hypercalcaemia
☐ B   Hyperkalaemia
☐ C   Hypocalcaemia
☐ D   Hypokalaemia
☐ E   Hyponatraemia

203 Which of the following electrolyte abnormalities increases the risk of digoxin toxicity?

☐ A   Hyperkalaemia
☐ B   Hypermagnesaemia

- C Hypernatraemia
- D Hypomagnesaemia
- E Hyponatraemia

204 Mrs H visits the accident and emergency department with symptoms of vomiting and confusion. Her lab results show she has low sodium levels. Which of the patient's medications could be causing this?

- A Estradiol 0.06% w/w gel, started 6 months ago
- B Ferrous sulfate 200mg OD, started 3 months ago
- C Lansoprazole 30mg OD, started 1 year ago
- D Paracetamol 500mg QDS, started 6 months ago
- E Sertraline 50mg OD, started 2 weeks ago

205 Which of the following preparations of iron can be administered parenterally?

- A Ferric carboxymaltose
- B Ferrous fumarate
- C Ferrous gluconate
- D Ferrous sulphate, dried
- E Ferrous sulphate

206 A 73-year-old male has been treated with a course of antibiotics. The patient is now complaining of a furred hairy tongue. Which of the following antibiotic is most likely responsible for this adverse effect?

- A Ciprofloxacin
- B Doxycycline
- C Flucloxacillin
- D Gentamicin
- E Metronidazole

207 A 48-year-old woman is newly diagnosed with urinary incontinence. She is started on solifenacin 5mg OD. Which of the following is the most appropriate counselling point?

☐ A Can affect performance of driving
☐ B Monitor blood pressure every 6 months
☐ C Monitor liver function tests every 6 months
☐ D Requires annual renal function monitoring
☐ E Take the first dose at night to avoid rebound hypotension

208 A 24 year-old-woman is newly diagnosed with irritable bowel syndrome (IBS). Her symptoms are predominantly abdominal cramps and constipation. She has tried self-management with lifestyle changes however, there has been minimal efficacy. The patient wishes to be started on pharmacological treatment. She does not take any concurrent medications and has no known drug allergies. Which of the following is the most appropriate treatment combination for this patient?

☐ A Alverine citrate and ispaghula husk
☐ B Amitriptyline and peppermint oil
☐ C Linaclotide and senna
☐ D Mebeverine hydrochloride and lactulose
☐ E Peppermint oil and loperamide

Questions 209 and 210 relate to the same patient.

209 A 36-year-old Caucasian man with a BMI of 38kg/m2 attends the weight loss management clinic. Which of the following classes is best described the patient's BMI?

☐ A Healthy weight
☐ B Overweight
☐ C Obesity Class I
☐ D Obesity Class II
☐ E Obesity Class III

210 Following a consultation at the obesity clinic, the patient is started on Saxenda® (liraglutide) subcutaneous injection as adjunct for obesity management. The patient has already participated in a weight management programme, which includes lifestyle changes, increased physical activity,

improved diet and eating behaviours. Which of the following points should be included whilst counselling the patient about naltrexone with bupropion?

☐ A   Risk of agranulocytosis
☐ B   Risk of dizziness
☐ C   Risk of liver failure
☐ D   Risk of postural hypotension
☐ E   Risk of suicide

Questions 211 to 213 relate to the same patient.

211 A 67-year-old man, who is admitted to the emergency department with upper gastrointestinal bleeding with oesopharyngeal varices. The patient has a background of alcohol dependence (50 units a week of lager), cirrhosis, gastro-oesophageal reflux disease, transient ischaemic attack (10 years ago) and familial hyperlipidaemia. He is currently taking the following medications:
- Clopidogrel tablet 75mg OD
- Lansoprazole capsule 30mg OD
- Disulfiram tablets 250mg OD
- Thiamine tablets 100mg OD
- Inclisiran subcutaneous injection 284mg every 6 months

In the acute management of this patient, which of the following medications should be withheld immediately?

☐ A   Clopidogrel
☐ B   Disulfiram
☐ C   Inclisiran
☐ D   Lansoprazole
☐ E   Thiamine

212 In the acute management of this patient, which of the following medications should be started?

☐ A   Andexanet alfa IV
☐ B   Famotidine PO

- C Pantoprazole IV
- D Terlipressin IV
- E Tranexamic acid PO

213 The patient underwent an ultrasound scan of the abdomen, which confirmed a diagnosis of portal hypertension. Which of the following medications should be started to prevent further episodes of oesophageal varices?

- A Amlodipine
- B Propranolol
- C Ramipril
- D Spironolactone
- E Verapamil

Questions 214 to 216 relate to the same patient.

214 A 45-year-old woman with a background of moderate Crohn's disease, who has been taking budesonide 3mg three times a day for the last four months. As the patient has been unable reduce the dose of budesonide whilst achieving remission, the gastroenterologist has suggested a trial of add-on therapy with azathioprine. Prior to starting azathioprine, which of the following pre-screenings should be performed?

- A Chest X-ray
- B Electrocardiogram (ECG)
- C Hepatitis screening
- D Thiopurine methyltransferase (TPMT) activity
- E Thyroid function tests (TFTs)

215 The pre-screening returns as unsatisfactory. As the patient is not suitable for azathioprine, the gastroenterologist has asked for your advice on an alternative treatment. Which of the following medications is the most suitable alternative to azathioprine?

- A Balsalazine
- B Infliximab

- C Methotrexate
- D Prednisolone
- E Vedolizumab

216 The patient's symptoms and condition did not respond despite adequate trialling period of the add-on therapy. At the latest review, her Crohn's disease is classified as severely active. Which of the following medications should be considered at this point?

- A Balslazine
- B Infliximab
- C Methotrexate
- D Prednisolone
- E Vedolizumab

217 A 70-year-old woman is diagnosed with *Helicobacter pylori* and requires eradication therapy. She has a background of hypertension and stroke (7 years ago) and is currently taking the following medications:
- Amlodipine tablet 10mg OD
- Clopidogrel tablet 75mg OD
- Atorvastatin 40mg OD

The patient has no known drug allergies. Which of the following combination for *Helicobacter pylori* eradication is most appropriate in this patient?
You may use the BNF treatment summary to help you: https://bnf.nice.org.uk/treatment-summaries/helicobacter-pylori-infection/

- A Amoxicillin, clarithromycin and lansoprazole for 7 days with no changes to the patient's regular medications.
- B Amoxicillin, metronidazole and famotidine for 7 days with no changes to the patient's regular medications.
- C Amoxicillin, metronidazole and lansoprazole for 7 days with no changes to the patient's regular medications.
- D Amoxicillin, metronidazole and omeprazole for 7 days with no changes to the patient's regular medications.
- E Clarithromycin, metronidazole and lansoprazole for 7 days with no changes to the patient's regular medications.

218 A 62-year-old man presents to the emergency department with upper abdominal pain. He undergoes further investigations which identify a gastric ulcer. Which of the following medications is most likely to be responsible for the finding?

- ☐ A Clopidogrel
- ☐ B Levothyroxine
- ☐ C Mirtazapine
- ☐ D Prednisolone
- ☐ E Tramadol

219 A 27-year-old woman with a background of complex Crohn's disease, has recently undergone surgical intervention resulting in an ileostomy. Which of the following formulations of medicine is not suitable for this patient?

- ☐ A Capsule
- ☐ B Enteric-coated tablet
- ☐ C Film-coated tablet
- ☐ D Liquid
- ☐ E Soluble tablet

220 A 54-year-old woman visits your community pharmacy requesting an over-the-counter treatment for sore throat. On further questioning, you gather that the patient also noticed unexplained bruises on her arms and legs which has appeared over the last week. The patient has a background of ulcerative colitis (currently in remission). Her PMR shows that the patient is taking the following medications from her GP:
- Octasa (mesalazine) tablet 1.2g OD
- Octasa (mesalazine) suppository 1g ON

Which of the following is the most appropriate advice to give to this patient?

- ☐ A Purchase over-the-counter products to manage her symptoms
- ☐ B See her GP as the dose of mesalazine may need to be increased
- ☐ C See her GP as the dose of mesalazine may need to be reduced

☐ D Stop taking/using mesalazine immediately and see her GP as soon as possible
☐ E The patient is experiencing a side effect of mesalazine, whilst it is safe to continue it, she may wish to see her GP for an alternative

221 You are the ward pharmacist and helping to update prescribing policies. The trainee doctor asks you if there are any monitoring requirements with oxybutynin. What should your advice be?

☐ A Monitor response to treatment at initial diagnosis and then annual specialist review.
☐ B Monitor the need for therapy every 4-6 weeks until symptoms stabilise and then every 6-12 months
☐ C Only monitor the need for therapy in children under the age of 5.
☐ D There is no routine recommended monitoring.
☐ E This medication is usually prescribed in elderly male patients, therefore monitor annually

222 You are the hospital pharmacist working on the gastroenterology unit. You are interpretating blood results. You find that their magnesium reading is 0.5mmol/L. Which of the following medicine is most likely causing this?

☐ A Cimetidine
☐ B Gaviscon
☐ C Lansoprazole
☐ D Misoprostol
☐ E Sando-K

223 You are the hospital pharmacist and reviewing Mr ZD (age 38 years), a patient who is undergoing treatment for peptic ulcer disease. Which of the following could be the cause of his admission?

☐ A Exercise
☐ B Long term NSAID use
☐ C Long term statin medication
☐ D Long term use of antihistamines
☐ E Overuse of short acting beta2 agonist inhalers

224 You are a prescriber working in primary care. Miss FO (age 28 years) presents with irritable bowel syndrome (IBS). She has abdominal discomfort which leads to episodes of diarrhoea and cramps. Her main concern today is the cramping - which of the following medications would be the most appropriate to issue?

- ☐ A Chlorphenamine
- ☐ B Docusate
- ☐ C Famotidine
- ☐ D Famotidine
- ☐ E Omeprazole

225 Which of the following medications should be promptly discontinued, and the patient should be instructed to consult their doctor if diarrhoea occurs?

- ☐ A Azathioprine
- ☐ B Clindamycin
- ☐ C Codeine
- ☐ D Magnesium trisilicate
- ☐ E Peppermint oil

226 Mrs AL (72 years) is diagnosed with osteoporosis following symptom review and also a DEXA scan at the fracture clinic. It is decided to initiate alendronic acid and adcal d3 caplets. Which of the following counselling points is the most relevant to her alendronic acid medication?

- ☐ A Take ONE 70mg tablet every day for 3 months
- ☐ B Take ONE 70mg tablet every day of the week apart from the day of taking adcal d3 caplets
- ☐ C Take ONE 70mg tablet every other day for 3 months
- ☐ D Take ONE 70mg tablet once a month
- ☐ E Take ONE 70mg tablet once a week

227 Mr FG (33years) is admitted onto a surgical ward following a upper gastrointestinal bleed. You are reviewing the medication chart. Which of the following medications would be most likely attributing to this gastro-intestinal bleed?

- [ ] A Cimetidine
- [ ] B Codeine
- [ ] C Gaviscon
- [ ] D Lansoprazole
- [ ] E Naproxen

228 Miss. AO a 24-year-old female visits your local pharmacy, and you diagnose her symptoms as primary dysmenorrhea. Which of the following statements is TRUE regarding primary dysmenorrhea?

- [ ] A Back pain is not an associated symptom
- [ ] B It is common for period pain to be caused by an underlying medical condition
- [ ] C Pain commences prior to the menstrual cycle
- [ ] D Pain should not occur during intercourse
- [ ] E The pain is often a sharp, shooting type of pain

229 Miss OP, a 25-year-old female, is in her first trimester of pregnancy. She has been experiencing suprapubic pain for the past four days along with a 'burning' sensation during urination. She takes no other medication and is well otherwise. Which of the following antibiotics is the most suitable for her condition?

- [ ] A Doxycycline 100mg daily for 5 days
- [ ] B Doxycycline 100mg daily for 7 days
- [ ] C Nitrofurantoin 100mg twice daily for 7 days
- [ ] D Trimethoprim 100mg daily for 3 days
- [ ] E Trimethoprim 100mg daily for 7 days

230 Following an uncomplicated urinary tract infection, Mrs FD (42 years) is prescribed nitrofurantoin 100mg twice daily for 3 days. You counsel her regarding potential side effects. Which of the following is MOST likely to occur?

- [ ] A Constipation
- [ ] B Dry mouth
- [ ] C Dysuria

☐ D Tremor
☐ E Urine may turn yellow or brown

Gastrointestinal medication (Questions 231 to 235).
For each clinical scenario below, choose the most appropriate medication from the list below. Each option can be used once, more than once, or not at all.

☐ A Bisacodyl
☐ B Hyoscine butylbromide
☐ C Lactulose
☐ D Lansoprazole
☐ E Mesalazine
☐ F Metoclopramide
☐ G Naloxegol
☐ H Ondansetron

231 A 48-year-old patient develops epigastric pain whilst taking naproxen, his GP would like to co-prescribe this medication to reduce the risk of gastro-intestinal side effects

232 A 32-year-old female patient has a history of irritable bowel syndrome (IBS). Her main concern is her abdominal cramping. Which is the most appropriate treatment?

233 A 58-year-old male patient takes co-dydramol regularly for his rheumatoid arthritis. Since taking his analgesia, he has developed constipation. His GP would like to initiate treatment for opioid induced constipation as he has previously trialled other laxatives which are not working effectively (fybogel and laxido).

234 Mr JS (28 years) has a history of ulcerative colitis. His specialist nurse would like to initiate treatment to manage his inflammatory condition and to reduce the number of flare ups. Renal function will be checked prior to initiation, at three months and then annually thereafter.

235 Miss TK (61 years) is undergoing chemotherapy for colon cancer. She is experiencing nausea and vomiting.

Blood and nutrition medication (Questions 236 to 240).
For each clinical scenario, choose the most appropriate medication from the list below. Each option can be used once, more than once, or not at all.

- ☐ A Colecalciferol
- ☐ B Ferinject
- ☐ C Ferrous sulphate
- ☐ D Folic acid
- ☐ E Hydroxocobalamin
- ☐ F Thiamine
- ☐ G Vitamin B Compound Strong
- ☐ H Vitamin B12 (Cyanocobalamin)

236 A patient is diagnosed with iron-deficiency anaemia following recent blood tests. She is 16 weeks pregnant, and the midwife would like to initiate treatment and repeat iron levels in 4 weeks.

237 A 29-year-old female patient is diagnosed with folate-deficient megaloblastic anaemia. The midwife recommends this medication to continue until term.

238 A 36-year-old male patient is admitted onto the admisisons medical unit due to alcohol dependence. The consultant prescribes him medication to detoxify the withdrawal symptoms. He is also prescribed parenteral treatment due to Wernicke's encephalopathy. He is discharged with oral medication to continue long term.

239 A 63-year- old female patient is diagnosed with pernicious anaemia (with no neurological involvement). This medication starts at 1mg 3 times a week for 2 weeks then will continue at 1mg every 3 months

240 A 38-year-old female patient is diagnosed with vitamin D deficiency and requires a high course 6-week treatment.

Immunosuppressant medication (Questions 241 to 245).
For each clinical scenario, choose the most appropriate medication from the list below. Each option can be used once, more than once, or not at all.

- [ ] A Azathioprine
- [ ] B Ciclosporin
- [ ] C Infliximab
- [ ] D Methotrexate
- [ ] E Mycophenolate
- [ ] F Prednisolone
- [ ] G Sulfasalazine
- [ ] H Tacrolimus

241 Mrs FN (64 years) is prescribed this medication for rheumatoid arthritis. It is a folic acid antagonist and requires routine blood level monitoring.

242 Mr ZN (age 24 years) is initiated topical treatment by his specialist for severe atopic eczema. He has previously not responded to conventional therapy

243 Mr LY (38 years) has recently undergone a kidney transplant. This immunosuppressant medication is prescribed as prophylaxis to prevent organ rejection. Monitoring consists of a full blood count every week for 4 weeks then twice a month for 2 months then every month in the first year.

244 Mrs LA (38 years) has rheumatoid arthritis but has not responded to DMARD therapy. Her consultant decides to initiate her on intravenous monoclonal antibodies.

245 Mr GC (47 years) is prescribed this medication for severe Crohn's disease. It is metabolised to mercaptopurine. Blood tests and monitoring for signs of myelosuppression are essential in long-term treatment.

Urinary symptoms (Questions 246 to 250).
For each clinical scenario, choose the most appropriate medication from the list below. Each option can be used once, more than once, or not at all.

- [ ] A Amitriptyline
- [ ] B Doxazosin
- [ ] C Finasteride
- [ ] D Mirabegron

- [ ] E Oxybutynin
- [ ] F Solifenacin
- [ ] G Tamsulosin
- [ ] H Trimethoprim

246 A 55-year-old male patient is initiated this medication to manage his urinary symptoms. It is advised to monitor his blood pressure due to his history of hypertension.

247 A 60-year-old male patient presents to the community pharmacy and would like treatment for his urinary symptoms. The pharmacist supplies a 6-week course and then advises GP review.

248 A 45-year-old patient is diagnosed with benign prostatic hyperplasia. He is prescribed a new medication and his partner is of childbearing potential. It is advised to use a condom is as the medication is excreted through semen.

249 A 58-year-old male patient is prescribed this medication for his lower urinary tract symptoms. It is an antimuscarinic and available in a patch formulation.

250 A 24-year-old female patient presents to the primary care centre with increased urinary frequency, dysuria and tiredness. She has tried over-the-counter cystitis sachets and found no benefit. A urine dipstick is actioned and shows raised leucocytes. The microbiology culture sample demonstrates a positive culture.

251 A 13-year-old male patient presents to the GP surgery with worsening asthma symptoms. He is currently prescribed Clenil 50 inhaler and a salbutamol inhaler (for PRN use). He is waking up at night with asthma symptoms. Which of the following is the most appropriate next step to consider?

- [ ] A Add low dose azithromycin (to be taken 3 times a week)
- [ ] B Add low dose prednisolone PO 5mg OD
- [ ] C Add montelukast and review in 6 weeks
- [ ] D Add salbutamol nebuliser therapy for night-time symptoms
- [ ] E Stop clenil and change to salmeterol

Respiratory medicines (Questions 252 to 256).
For each clinical scenario, choose the most appropriate medication from the list below. Each option can be used once, more than once, or not at all.

☐ A Beclometasone
☐ B Ipratropium
☐ C Montelukast
☐ D Prednisolone
☐ E Roflumilast
☐ F Salbutamol
☐ G Theophylline
☐ H Tiotropium

252 An 18-year-old female patient is suffering with asthma symptoms. She is currently using her short acting inhaler and has a relatively new diagnosis (diagnosed 4 weeks ago) but is continuing to struggle with her daily activities and struggling to sleep at night. Her GP recommends this as the next step in her treatment plan.

253 Overuse of this medication can lead to tremors, shakes and hypokalaemia.

254 Mr WN (69 years) has severe chronic obstructive pulmonary disease which is currently poorly controlled. His respiratory consultant decides to start him on a phosphodiesterase type-4 inhibitor due to its anti-inflammatory properties.

255 Mr TJ (57 years) is newly diagnosed with chronic obstructive pulmonary disease following a 21-year smoking pack history. He requires a long-acting bronchodilator for long term maintenance treatment.

256 Mr DP (48 years) has chronic asthma and prescribed this medication for preventative treatment. A dose adjustment is required as he stopped smoking 3 weeks ago

Low weighted questions

257 Miss N, aged 25, presents to the pharmacy with a concern regarding her eyes. Upon discussion, you find that she has been experiencing dryness in both eyes after being newly started on some medication. Which of the following medications is most likely to have caused her new eye condition?

- ☐ A Amitriptyline
- ☐ B Aspirin
- ☐ C Metformin
- ☐ D Mirtazapine
- ☐ E Sulfasalazine

258 Mrs MJ, aged 36, presents in the pharmacy with a unilateral red eye. The patient tells you it is quite painful and upon examination you find that she has an irregularly shaped pupil. Which of the following conditions is the patient most likely to be suffering?

- ☐ A Bacterial conjunctivitis
- ☐ B Keratitis
- ☐ C Subconjunctival haemorrhage
- ☐ D Uveitis
- ☐ E Viral conjuctivitis

259 A 30-year-old woman with multiple myeloma is treated with IV melphalan injection. Seven day after receiving melphalan, the patient presents at emergency department with fever, sore throat, vomitting, generalised muscle and joint pain. Which of the following courses of action must be performed as a priority?

- ☐ A Administer broad-spectrum antibacterial therapy according to local guidance
- ☐ B Administer broad-spectrum antibacterial therapy according to NICE guidance

- C Administer IV paracetamol to reduce the fever
- D Take a blood sample for culture
- E Take a blood sample to check full blood count

260 Which of the following chemotherapy must not be administered intrathecally?

- A Cytarabine
- B Etoposide
- C Methotrexate
- D Mitomycin
- E Vincristine

261 A 75-year-old man has been diagnosed with high-risk localised prostate cancer. He is treated with radical radiotherapy in combination with androgen deprivation therapy. Which of the following is a side effect of androgen deprivation therapy?

- A Enteropathy
- B Gynaecomastia
- C Meningioma
- D Osteoporosis
- E Tumour flare

262 A 60-year-old woman with T1c human epidermal growth factor receptor 2 (HER2) positive invasive breast cancer is treated with a combination of trastuzumab and surgery. When counselling the patient about trastuzumab, which of the following points should be included?

- A Risk of cardiac dysfunction
- B Risk of ketoacidosis
- C Risk of liver failure
- D Risk of peripheral neuropathy
- E Risk of renal failure

263 A 55-year-old woman has recently been diagnosed with oestrogen-receptor positive invasive breast cancer. The patient is post-menopausal

and is at high risk of disease recurrence. What is the first line endocrine therapy for this patient?

☐ A Goserelin
☐ B Letrozole
☐ C Pertuzumab
☐ D Tamoxifen
☐ E Zoledronic acid

Question 264 to 266 relate to the same patient.

264 A 50-year-old man attends your clinic with a painful and swollen big toe joint. This is his first episode, and his symptoms have been present for over a month. Blood results show a urate level of 574micromol/litre which confirms a diagnosis of gout. All other blood results are within normal range. The patient has a history of asthma and type II diabetes. He is currently taking the following medications:
- Fostair 100/6 inhaler (MART regimen)
- Metformin MR 2g OD

Which of the following treatments is most appropriate for this patient's acute gout attack?

☐ A Anakinra
☐ B Colchicine
☐ C Febuxostat
☐ D Naproxen with lansoprazole
☐ E Prednisolone

265 Following the acute attack, the patient is started on allopurinol for long term prophylaxis of gout. Select the most appropriate timescale for this patient to start his allopurinol.

☐ A Immediately after the flare
☐ B 3-5 days after the flare
☐ C 5-7 days after the flare
☐ D 7-14 days after the flare
☐ E 14-28 days after the flare

266 The patient's dose of allopurinol is up-titrated without any side effects or concerns. At his annual medication review, the patient reports no further acute flare ups. There is no tophi present. You perform a blood test to check the patient's urate level. Which of the following is the correct target urate level for this patient?

☐ A 260mmol/L
☐ B 300mmol/L
☐ C 310mmol/L
☐ D 360mmol/L
☐ E 400mmol/L

267 A 57-year-old woman attends your minor ailment clinic with mild dry eyes. On history taking, you gather that the main symptoms are dry sensation in the eyes which has been present for over two weeks; there is no pain and her vision is not affected. She wears glasses but does not use contact lenses. The patient also has hypothyroidism and takes levothyroxine 125microgram once daily in the morning. She works as a nurse and due to her shift working pattern, the patient wishes to have a treatment with minimal application frequency. Which of the following preparations is most appropriate for this patient?

☐ A Carbomer eye gel
☐ B Carmellose eye drops
☐ C Hypromellose eye drops
☐ D Paraffin containing eye ointment
☐ E Sodium hyaluronate eye drops

268 A 64-year-old man who is newly diagnosed with chronic open-angle glaucoma is awaiting 360 selective laser trabeculoplasty. In the interim, the ophthalmologist has recommended topical treatment with a prostaglandin analogue. Which of the following is a prostaglandin analogue?

☐ A Apraclonidine
☐ B Bimatoprost
☐ C Brimonidine

- D Dorzolamide
- E Levobunolol

269 A 34-year-old woman with a background of monoarthritis received Cimzia® (certolizumab pegol) throughout her pregnancy. She gave birth a week ago and she is not breastfeeding. At which age would it be safe for the newborn baby to be given live attenuated vaccine?

- A 4 weeks
- B 2 months
- C 6 months
- D 9 months
- E 12 months

270 A 20-year-old man gives consent to receive primary COVID-19 vaccination at your pharmacy. You administer a dose of Corminaty® 30micrograms into the patient's deltoid without any adverse effects. The patient is not immunosuppressed and does not require rapid immunisation. What is the minimum interval between the two doses of COVID-19 vaccination in this case?

- A 4 weeks
- B 6 weeks
- C 8 weeks
- D 10 weeks
- E 12 weeks

271 A 57-year-old man is in theatre for a cholecystectomy. During the intubation sequence, the patient goes into anaphylactic shock. Which of the following drug is most likely to be responsible?

- A Fentanyl
- B Ketamine
- C Parecoxib
- D Propofol
- E Suxamethonium

272 A 56-year-old woman is undergoing a cystoscopy and receives an injection of botulinum toxin into the bladder for detrusor instability. Which of the following best describes the therapeutic effect of botulinum toxin?

☐ A Antagonism of achetylcholine at the post junctional receptor
☐ B Increased neuronal reuptake of achetylcholine
☐ C Inhibition of acetylcholine release
☐ D Inhibition of acetylcholine reuptake
☐ E Potentiation of acetylcholinesterase

273 An 8-year-old boy with adrenocortical insufficiency is prescribed mineralocorticoid replacement therapy. Which of the following corticosteroids is most suitable for this patient's mineralocorticoid replacement therapy?

☐ A Betamethasone
☐ B Dexamethasone
☐ C Fludrocortisone
☐ D Methylprednisolone
☐ E Prednisolone

274 A 14-year-old girl presents at your minor ailment clinic with her parents. The presenting complaint is symptoms of acute sinusitis for 2 weeks. The parents reports that she has not yet tried any over-the-counter treatment and there has been no improvements in the symptoms so far. The patient has no other medical conditions and there is no allergies or intolerance. Select the most appropriate course of action to manage this case.

☐ A Antibacterial therapy according to local guidance
☐ B Nasal fluticasone for 7 days
☐ C Nasal mometasone furoate for 14 days
☐ D Paracetamol OTC for management of pain and fever
☐ E Self-care advice

275 A 13-year-old boy, accompanied by his parents, presents at your pharmacy with functional constipation. On further questioning, you identify that he has experienced constipation for over two weeks and there is no faecal

impaction. His diet comprises of mainly fast food and fizzy drinks. He is not taking any other medications and has no other medical condition. Select the most appropriate management option in this case.

☐ A Offer advice on diet modification and adequate fluid intake
☐ B Offer OTC treatment with docusate sodium and advice on diet modification
☐ C Offer OTC treatment with lactulose and advice on diet modification
☐ D Offer OTC treatment with macrogol and advice on diet modification
☐ E Refer the patient back to their GP for management

276 A 12-year-old girl presents at the paediatric emergency department with an unintentional acute overdose of propranolol. The child is in cardiogenic shock and a bolus dose of glucagon injection has been administered. The child weighs 50kg. What dose of glucagon should be administered next?

The BNFc monograph for glucagon is provided here: https://bnfc.nice.org.uk/drugs/glucagon/

☐ A 1mg over 1 minute
☐ B 2.5mg over 1 minute
☐ C 7.5mg over 1 minute
☐ D 1mg per hour infusion
☐ E 2.5mg per hour infusion

277 A 9-year-old boy requires ibuprofen for the relief of pain associated with a sprained ankle during a football game. The child weighs 30kg. What is the most appropriate dose of ibuprofen to be administered every eight hours?

The BNFc monograph for ibuprofen is provided here: https://bnfc.nice.org.uk/drugs/ibuprofen/

☐ A 50mg
☐ B 100mg
☐ C 150mg
☐ D 200mg
☐ E 400mg

278 A 15-year-old girl attends your clinic with her mother to discuss starting hormonal contraception. The patient reports her menarche occurred at 13 years. She is currently not sexually active and states that she is not intending to become so. The mother wishes for her child to be started on hormonal contraception 'just in case'. Which of the following approaches is most appropriate in this case?

☐ A As the patient is under 16-years old, you must carry out the consultation with mother in the child's best interest
☐ B As the patient is under 16-years-old, you must follow criteria set out in Fraser guidelines
☐ C As the patient is under 16-years-old, it is good practice for you to follow criteria set out in Fraser guidelines
☐ D As the patient is under 16-years-old, you must assess if she is Gillick competent
☐ E As the patient is under 16-years-old, it is good practice for you to assess if she is Gillick competent

279 A 6-year-old boy presents at your community pharmacy with his mother to seek your advice about scabies. The mother is concerned as there has been a scabies outbreak at school. On reviewing the child, you note there is a red rash with intense itching and signs of burrow on the skin. A diagnosis of scabies is made. Which of the following statement is correct about scabies treatment?

☐ A Crotamiton is a suitable treatment to manage itching associated with scabies
☐ B It is not necessary to treat all members of the household simultaneously
☐ C Malathion, permethrin and benzyl benzoate are suitable treatment for scabies in children
☐ D Permethrin should be applied after a hot bath to increase its efficacy
☐ E Malathion should be applied daily for 3 consecutive doses

280 A 68-year-old man with a background of type II diabetes and obesity (Body Mass Index of 35 kg/m2), and is currently on the following medications:

- Atorvastatin 20mg once a day
- Metformin modified-release 1gram twice a day
- Ozempic (semaglutide) 0.5mg subcutaneous injection once weekly
- Pioglitazone 45mg once a day

The patient presents at your community pharmacy and complains of increased urinary frequency, burning pain upon urination and presence of blood in urine. The symptoms have been present for two weeks and is worsening. Which of the following is the most appropriate advice to give to this patient?

- ☐ A The symptoms described could be a side effect of metformin. The patient should stop taking metformin immediately and arrange an appointment with the GP as soon as possible.
- ☐ B The symptoms described could be a side effect of Ozempic® (semaglutide) subcutaneous injection. The patient should stop taking Ozempic® (semaglutide) subcutaneous injection immediately and arrange an appointment with the GP as soon as possible.
- ☐ C The symptoms described could be a side effect of pioglitazone. The patient should stop taking pioglitazone immediately and arrange an appointment with the GP as soon as possible.
- ☐ D The symptoms described could be a urinary tract infection, which can be associated with type II diabetes. The patient should book an appointment with the GP for a course of antibiotic.
- ☐ E The symptoms described could be due to his uncontrolled type II diabetes. The patient should book an appointment with the GP to have his dose of Ozempic (semaglutide) subcutaneous injection increased as soon as possible.

281 A 28-year-old woman presents at your community pharmacy with a prescription for sodium valproate. This is her first dispensing of this medication. Which of the following statements is correct in relation to sodium valproate?

- ☐ A If sodium valproate is stopped, it is advisable to discontinue the treatment immediately

☐ B If used for epilepsy, the patient must remain on the same brand of sodium valproate
☐ C It is safe for the patient to fall pregnant whilst taking sodium valproate
☐ D Pre-treatment monitoring of sodium valproate include liver function test and full blood count
☐ E Sodium valproate in licensed in the treatment of epilepsy, mania and prophylaxis of migraine

282 You are a pharmacist working in General Practice. When conducting an audit into the prescribing of hormonal replacement therapy in menopausal and post-menopausal women, you identify a prescribing error where a woman with an intact uterus has been unintentionally prescribed unopposed oestrogen for six months. You report the incident using the practice incident reporting system and conduct a root cause analysis to identify the contributing factors to the incident. You refer the patient to the General Practitioner (GP) for a follow-up and an ultrasound scan is arranged. The patient is prescribed progestogen therapy alongside oestrogen. A formal apology letter is sent to the patient from the practice. Which of the following GPhC's *Standards for Pharmacy Professionals* is best demonstrated in this example?

☐ A Pharmacy professionals must behave in a professional manner
☐ B Pharmacy professionals must demonstrate leadership
☐ C Pharmacy professionals must provide person-centred care
☐ D Pharmacy professionals must respect duty of candour
☐ E Pharmacy professionals must speak up when they have concerns or when things go wrong

283 A patient comes to your community pharmacy as the pharmacy recently dispensed medication for them. They report an adverse reaction. You note it is a new drug on the market under the black triangle scheme. It is important for pharmacists to report adverse reactions to which organisation?

☐ A GPhC
☐ B MHRA
☐ C National Institute of Clinical Excellence

- D Pharmacist Defence Association
- E Royal Pharmaceutical Society

284 You are a community pharmacist and receive a prescription for lorazepam. The trainee pharmacy technician asks you about classification of medicines drugs. Which of the following is the correct classification of lorazepam?

- A Pharmacy medicine
- B Prescription only medicine
- C Schedule 2 CD
- D Schedule 3 CD
- E Schedule 4 Part 1 CD

285 Mr GZ (aged 51 years) contacts the community pharmacy at which you work. He reports his soft contact lenses as frequently changing colour. Which of the following medicines is most likely to have caused this?

- A Ramipril
- B Rifampicin
- C Rifaximin
- D Riluzole
- E Rizatriptan

286 You are the responsible pharmacist in the local community pharmacy. Mr GV (19 years old) was dispensed phenoxymethylpenicillin for his tonsillitis. Mr GV confirms he has no allergies. The following day, he returns to the pharmacy with concerns about a rash he has developed. He reports no other symptoms however his throat pain continues to persist. What course of action would you take?

- A Advise him to contact an urgent care centre
- B Advise him to contact 999
- C Advise him to contact his GP today
- D Advise him to continue with the medication as the side effects are transient
- E Dispense a suitable alternative

Law (Questions 287 to 291).
For each scenario, choose the most appropriate duration from the list below. Each option can be used once, more than once, or not at all.

☐ A Daily
☐ B 72 hours
☐ C 5 days
☐ D Weekly
☐ E 28 days
☐ F 30 days
☐ G 3 months
☐ H 6 months

287 The maximum validity of a prescription for tramadol.

288 An EEA prescriber must write a prescription within this time frame following an emergency supply.

289 The maximum validity of a prescription for 100mls of morphine sulfate 10mg/5ml.

290 The maximum validity of a prescription for pregabalin.

291 The maximum number of days that can be supplied of a prescription only medicine, which is not a controlled drug, for an emergency supply at the request of a patient.

292 Pregnancy prevention programmes protect females of childbearing potential by minimising the risk of becoming pregnant while taking certain medication. Which of the following does NOT apply to sodium valproate?

☐ A A patient card should be provided each time the medication is dispensed
☐ B Ensure a patient information leaflet is provided each time the medication is dispensed
☐ C Ensure the dispensing label does not cover the warning label

- D Under the PPP, prescriptions are only valid for 7 days
- E Valproate preparations should be dispensed in original packs whenever possible

293 Which of the following statements regarding veterinary medicines is incorrect?

- A A written prescription is not required for a category NFA-VPS medicine
- B For prescriptions for schedule 2 and 3 controlled drugs the RCVS registration number of the prescriber is required
- C Prescriptions are valid for 28 days from the appropriate date
- D Records for POM-V and POM-VPS products must be kept for at least 5 years
- E The name and address of the prescribing veterinary surgeon must appear on the dispensing label

294 Which of the following activities can take place without the supervision of a pharmacist?

- A Handing checked prescriptions to patients
- B Handing checked prescriptions to the delivery driver
- C Processing waste stock medicines or patient retuned medicines
- D Sale or supply of P medicines
- E Wholesale of medicines

295 You are a community pharmacist and are asked to supply some medicine at the request of a prescriber. Which of the following does NOT need to be included in the POM register entry?

- A Information on the nature of the emergency
- B The date on the prescription
- C The date the POM was supplied
- D The name and address of the prescriber
- E The quantity supplied

296 Which of the following controlled drugs cannot be prescribed by a physiotherapist independent prescriber?

☐ A Fentanyl patches
☐ B Morphine for injection
☐ C Oral diazepam
☐ D Oral morphine
☐ E Oxycodone for injection

297 Mr H, a 42-year-old man, comes into your pharmacy asking to purchase orlistat to help him lose weight. Which of the following statements regarding orlistat is NOT correct?

☐ A 60mg of orlistat should be taken 3 times a day
☐ B It is contraindicated in patients who take warfarin
☐ C It is only for use in adults 18 or over
☐ D Orlistat should be taken with a low-fat and mildly hypocaloric diet
☐ E Treatment should not exceed 9 months

298 Mr T, aged 23, visits the pharmacy with a concern about his feet. He tells you his left foot is very itchy and upon examination the skin between his toes looks red and flaky. He says that the itchiness keeps him up at night. Which OTC product would Mr T benefit from the most?

☐ A Canesten® Athletes foot 1% w/w cream (clotrimazole 1% w/w)
☐ B Daktacort® hydrocortisone cream (miconazole 2% w/w/ hydrocortisone 1% w/w)
☐ C Daktarin® intensive cream (ketoconazole 2% w/w)
☐ D Lamisil® AT 1% cream (terbinafine 1% w/w)
☐ E Mycota® powder (zinc undecylenate 20% w/w/undecylenic acid 2% w/w)

299 Miss E, aged 19, visits the pharmacy and wants something to treat a verruca on her foot. She takes insulin for type 1 diabetes. Which of the following is most appropriate for this patient?

☐ A Refer to GP
☐ B Supply a cryotherapy kit
☐ C Supply OTC Bazuka®
☐ D Supply OTC salicylic acid
☐ E Supply verruca plasters

300 In which of the following cases can sumatriptan (Migraitan®) be supplied OTC?

☐ A A history of five migraine attacks occurring over a period of one year
☐ B A patient taking amitriptyline
☐ C Headaches lasting over 24 hours
☐ D History of seizures
☐ E Patients with hypertension

301 Miss MA (age 26 years) presents to the pharmacy with lower back pain. She uses a salbutamol inhaler to control her asthma. Which of the following is the least appropriate painkiller to supply?

☐ A Nurofen® plus
☐ B Panadol®
☐ C Panadol® Extra
☐ D Paramol®
☐ E Solpadeine®

302 Miss H visits the pharmacy to buy paracetamol syrup for her five-year-old child who has a fever along with flu like symptoms. The child has no other medical conditions. Which of the following is the most appropriate dose to be administered every 6 hours?

☐ A 60mg
☐ B 120mg
☐ C 180mg
☐ D 240mg
☐ E 375mg

303 Which of the following pieces of advice regarding the self-care of chickenpox is the LEAST appropriate?

☐ A Chlorphenamine can be used to relieve itch in patients over the age of 1
☐ B Increase fluid intake to avoid dehydration
☐ C Paracetamol or ibuprofen can be used to reduce fever or pain
☐ D Topical calamine lotion can be used to relieve itch
☐ E Wear clothes made from smooth cotton fabric

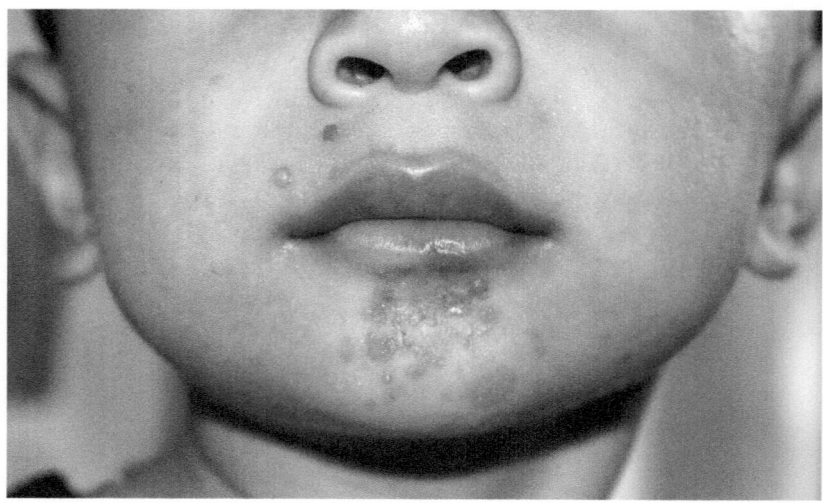

Source: Shutterstock.com

304 Miss G, presents at the pharmacy with her 4-year-old child. The child has red fluid filled bumps around his mouth as shown above. Which of the following conditions is the child most likely to have?

- ☐ A Chickenpox
- ☐ B Impetigo
- ☐ C Measles
- ☐ D Scarlet fever
- ☐ E Shingles

305 Which one of the following is NOT a characteristic of scarlet fever?

- ☐ A Aching fingers, wrists or knees
- ☐ B Sandpaper-like rash
- ☐ C Sore throat
- ☐ D Swollen neck glands
- ☐ E White coating on the tongue

306 Which of the following is NOT a standard for pharmacy professionals?

- ☐ A Demonstrate leadership

☐ B Maintain, develop and use their professional knowledge and skills
☐ C Speak up when things go wrong
☐ D Use professional judgment
☐ E Work independently

307 All GPhC registered professionals must complete their revalidation records each year. For this, they may carry out a range of CPD activities relevant to their practice. Which of the following standards apply to the statement above?

☐ A Behave in a professional manner
☐ B Demonstrate Leadership
☐ C Maintain, develop and use their professional knowledge and skills
☐ D Provide patient centred care
☐ E Use professional judgement

308 Which of the following is an example of patient centred care?

☐ A Pharmacy professionals have the information they need to provide appropriate care
☐ B Pharmacy professionals maintain appropriate personal and professional boundaries
☐ C Pharmacy professionals practise only when fit to do so
☐ D Pharmacy professionals recognise and work within the limits of their knowledge and skills, and refer to others when needed
☐ E Pharmacy professionals recognise their own values and beliefs but do not impose them on other people

309 Pharmacists must understand the importance of managing information responsibly and securely, and apply this to their practice. Which professional standard is this relevant to?

☐ A Behave in a professional manner
☐ B Communicate effectively
☐ C Demonstrate leadership
☐ D Respect and maintain the person's confidentiality and privacy
☐ E Use professional judgment

310 Which of the following vaccines is recommended in patients with a history of splenectomy?

☐ A Hepatitis A vaccine
☐ B Hepatitis B vaccine
☐ C Hepatitis C vaccine
☐ D Pneumococcal vaccine
☐ E Rabies vaccine

311 You are advising a prescriber about the treatment for uncomplicated uncomplicated chlamydia trachomatis urethritis. You have access to the SPC. https://www.medicines.org.uk/emc/product/6541/smpc
You advise the correct treatment is?

☐ A Azithromycin 1 g once daily for 1 day
☐ B Azithromycin 500mg once daily for 3 days
☐ C Azithromycin 500mg on day 1, 250mg on day 2
☐ D Azithromycin 500mg on day 1, 250mg on day 2 to day 5
☐ E Azithromycin 500mg on day 1, 250mg on day 2 to day 7

312 A community nurse seeks your advice and asks what the most appropriate vaccine is, for a newborn infant who resides in an area of high tuberculosis. Which would be the most appropriate vaccine?

☐ A BCG vaccine
☐ B COVID vaccine
☐ C Influenza vaccine
☐ D MenB vaccine
☐ E Pneumococcal vaccine

313 Miss DL (22 years) would like to buy over the counter paracetamol for her 3 year old daughter. A suitable paracetamol dose for her daughter is?

☐ A 60 mg every 4–6 hours; maximum 4 doses per day
☐ B 120 mg every 4–6 hours; maximum 4 doses per day
☐ C 120 mg every 2–3 hours; maximum 6 doses per day
☐ D 180 mg every 4–6 hours; maximum 4 doses per day
☐ E 180 mg every 2–3 hours; maximum 6 doses per day

314 You are the regular community pharmacist at your local branch. Miss PA (31 years) would like to discuss her oral contraception medication with you. She is currently taking Microgynon® 30 ED tablets. She is concerned her compliance is not good and would like to discuss appropriate options for her. She confirms unprotected sexual intercourse has not taken place. Which of the following is a correct statement?

☐ A Consider switching treatment to a patch
☐ B Refer to family planning services
☐ C Refer to the sexual health clinic
☐ D Supply over the counter EllaOne®
☐ E Supply over the counter Levonelle®

Eye conditions (Questions 315 to 318).
For each clinical scenario, choose the most appropriate medication from the list below. Each option can be used once, more than once, or not at all.

☐ A Bacterial conjunctivitis
☐ B Blepharitis
☐ C Dry eye
☐ D Keratitis
☐ E Scleritis
☐ F Subconjunctival haemorrhage
☐ G Uveitis
☐ H Viral conjunctivitis

315 Self-limiting red eye condition which usually occurs due to a burst vessel. The condition will resolve itself in 1-2 weeks.

316 Usually affects patients bilaterally. Symptoms include eye irritation, itching, or discomfort. Blurry vision and watery eyes also occur. Management includes using artificial gel tears if lifestyle measures do not provide relief.

317 Inflammation of the eye lids which appear red, swollen or sore. Both eyes are affected, usually worse on a morning. Symptoms can be managed with self-care measures such as eyelid hygiene and warm, compression. Regular

cleaning of the eye and avoiding irritants is also effective. If self care measures are ineffective then topical or oral antibiotics can be prescribed.

318 A patient presents to the community pharmacy with unilateral purulent discharge, there is crusting of the lids and this was stuck together on waking. You advise the patient the condition is self limiting however the patient would prefer over the counter treatment in the form of topical antibiotics.

Ear, nose and throat (Questions 319 to 321).
For each clinical scenario, choose the most appropriate management plan from the list below. Each option can be used once, more than once, or not at all.

- ☐ A Amoxicillin capsules
- ☐ B Beclometasone nasal spray
- ☐ C Benzydamine oral spray
- ☐ D Earcalm® spray
- ☐ E Olive oil ear drops
- ☐ F Otomize® ear spray
- ☐ G Pheonxymethylpenicillin tablets
- ☐ H Refer to A&E

319 A 3-year-old patient presents to the GP surgery with neck pain, fever, muffled voice, a displaced uvula. The present with an enlarged, displaced tonsil (the patient has a muffled voice) and there is also swelling noted.

320 A 23-year-old patient presents to the community pharmacy with a sore throat. She has recently had a cough, flu-like symptoms and a fever. She is worried about her upcoming university examinations.

321 A 52-year-old patient presents with one sided ear discomfort. He has noted a blocked / fullness feeling. You examine the ear and unable to view the tympanic membrane.

Skin (Questions 322 to 326).
For each clinical scenario, choose the most appropriate management plan from the list below. Each option can be used once, more than once, or not at all.

- ☐ A Clobetasone butyrate 0.05% cream
- ☐ B Clotrimazole 1% cream
- ☐ C Clotrimazole 2% cream
- ☐ D Hydrocortisone 1% cream
- ☐ E Ketoconazole 2% shampoo
- ☐ F Mometasone furoate 1% cream
- ☐ G Permethrin 5% cream
- ☐ H Terbinafine 1% cream

322 A patient is diagnosed with scabies, this medication is issued to treat symptoms affecting the whole body.

323 A 12-year-old patient is diagnosed with an insect bite following their recent travels abroad. This can be supplied by a community pharmacist.

324 A patient is diagnosed with seborrhoeic dermatitis.

325 A moderate potency steroid based cream.

326 A potent steroid based cream.

327 A 17-year-old presents in the pharmacy asking to discuss an issue with their eye. The patient advises you that their eye has been watery and there is a yellow sticky discharge. This is worst on waking, but the gritty feeling in the eye is causing discomfort. The patient's vision has not been affected and there is no pain within the eye; but they are keen to get it treated as they are due to attend a party and want to look their best as soon as possible. What is the most appropriate course of action?

- ☐ A Advise the patient that these symptoms will pass in a few days - do not sell anything
- ☐ B Refer to GP
- ☐ C Refer to the Eye Hospital
- ☐ D Sell chloramphenicol 0.5% eye drops
- ☐ E Sell sodium cromoglycate 2% eye drops

328 A patient purchases some eye drops to treat bacterial conjunctivitis and is given chloramphenicol 0.5% eye drops. Which of the following is the appropriate method of storing the drops during treatment?
The SPC is provided here: https://www.medicines.org.uk/emc/product/427/smpc#gref

- ☐ A Store at room temperature and discard seven days after opening
- ☐ B Store in a cool dark cupboard- out of the reach of children, discard 28 days after opening
- ☐ C Store in a refrigerator between 2-8°C and discard after 28 days from opening
- ☐ D Store in a refrigerator between 2-8°C and discard when expiry date on bottle is reached
- ☐ E Store in a refrigerator until use then store at room temperature for seven days after opening

329 A 55-year-old patient visits the pharmacy and asks for advice regarding a cold sore that appeared on their bottom lip yesterday. The patient states that this occurred previously, about 7 months ago but it healed naturally and they did not treat it at that occurrence. Since the patient has a big event to attend in a few days, they want to purchase something that will speed up the healing of the lesion. Which of the following products is the most appropriate to supply top treat the patient's cold sore?

- ☐ A Blistex® Relief cream
- ☐ B Bonjela®
- ☐ C Carmex® Classic Moisturising Lip Balm
- ☐ D Petroleum jelly
- ☐ E Zovirax® cream (aciclovir 5% cream)

330 A 60-year-old patient presents to a community pharmacy after feeling unwell for the last few days. They developed a urine infection two days ago which means they are urinating frequently. You need to consider if the patient may be suffering from sepsis. Which one of the following symptoms is NOT a symptom of sepsis?

- ☐ A Confusion or disorientation

- B Dry gritty eyes
- C Fever, shivering or feeling cold
- D Severe breathlessness
- E Skin rash that does not fade when pressed with a glass

331 One of your regular customers comes to the pharmacy to purchase some hydrocortisone cream to manage their eczema which has flared up on their hands. They have had eczema for many years and usually obtain their hydrocortisone on prescription from their GP but there are no available appointments so they decided to purchase some instead. The eczema has affected their ankles, shins and hands; the skin on their hands is cracked and weeping. Which is the best course of action to take for this patient?

- A Advise to moisturise with an emollient and to stop all steroid treatments
- B Refer to GP
- C Refer to walk-in-centre
- D Sell clobetasone cream to manage eczema
- E Sell hydrocortisone 1% cream to manage eczema

332 A mother presents to the pharmacy asking you about some symptoms their child is suffering from. The 26-month-old child has been complaining about itching and has been scratching their bottom a lot, something the child has not done before. On changing the child's nappy, the mum has seen some white or cream coloured thread-like objects in the faeces. You diagnose threadworms and decide to supply mebendazole. Which of the following statements regarding the over-the-counter sale of mebendazole is correct?

- A Mebendazole dose needs to be repeated after five days to prevent reinfection
- B Mebendazole is administered rectally for the best effect
- C Mebendazole is licensed is children over 3 years old
- D Mebendazole is safe to take in pregnancy
- E It is strongly recommended that all members of the family are treated at the same time

Over-the-counter (OTC) medicines (Questions 333 to 341).
For each of the following medicines, choose the most appropriate age from the list below. Each option can be used once, more than once, or not at all.

☐ A 4 months
☐ B 2 years
☐ C 10 years
☐ D 12 years
☐ E 16 years
☐ F 18 years
☐ G 45 years
☐ H 65 years

333 The minimum age you can supply OTC sumatriptan.

334 The minimum age you can supply OTC hydrocortisone cream.

335 The minimum age you can supply OTC fluconazole 150mg capsules.

336 The minimum age you can supply OTC Sudafed decongestant tablets.

337 The minimum age you can supply OTC amorolfine.

338 The minimum age you can supply OTC oral miconazole gel.

339 The minimum age you can supply OTC mebendazole.

340 The minimum age you can supply tamsulosin.

341 The minimum age you can supply a 2% external clotrimazole cream and 500mg clotrimazole pessary.

Calculations questions

342 Drug Z has a half-life of 5 hours. The initial plasma level of the drug is 6000mg/L. What will the plasma level be after 12 hours.

☐ A 3000mg/L
☐ B 1500mg/L
☐ C 1200mg/L
☐ D 1050mg/L
☐ E 750mg/L

343 Miss M is prescribed a 10 day course of high dose prednisolone for an episode of Bell's palsy. The dosage instructions are as follows:

'take 60mg once daily for the first five days, then reduced by 10mg every day until the course is completed'

How many prednisolone 5mg tablets would you need to dispense this prescription?

☐ A 42
☐ B 84
☐ C 90
☐ D 100
☐ E 168

344 You are reviewing prescribing habits as a way of reducing medication costs. Currently the first line treatment for urinary tract infections is nitrofurantoin 100mg MR caps, 1 capsule BD 5/7 but you are looking to suggest that this changed to nitrofurantoin 100mg tablets, 1 tablet BD 5/7 instead. The cost of both drugs are as follows:
- Nitrofurantoin MR caps 100 x 14 cost £9.75
- Nitrofurantoin 100mg tablets x 28 cost £3.00

Calculate how money can be saved if 150 patients in the region are switched in the future. Give your answer to the nearest £5 Great British Pounds

345 A patient weighing 78kg has been admitted to hospital to manage oedema caused by cardiac disease. They have been prescribed a continuous furosemide infusion at a rate of 0.75mg/kg over a 60 minute period. Furosemide 10mg/1mL infusion is available and is to be given at rate of no more than 4mg per minute. How many micrograms/min does the patient receive each minute of the infusion?

346 You are working as a pharmacist in a compounding laboratory and have been tasked to produce a batch of diazepam suppositories due to long term supply issues affecting diazepam rectal tubes. Your order is for 175 diazepam 2g suppositories, each containing 5mg of active substance in a theobroma oil base. If diazepam has a DV of 1.5, how many grams of theobroma oil is needed? Do not calculate for excess. Give your answer to 2 decimal places.

347 You receive a prescription from the outpatient endocrinology clinic for a 0.8 % estradiol ointment using white soft paraffin as a base. You need to make 600g of this preparation. How many milligrams of estradiol powder is required to prepare this item?

348 A patient weighing 72kg has developed pyelonephritis and been admitted to hospital for treatment. The patient has been prescribed one vial of co-amoxiclav 1000/200mg solution for injection TDS for 5 days. The sodium content of each vial is 2.7mmol. The RMM of sodium is 23 g/mol. The patient's sodium levels are found to be raised so the medical team would like you to calculate the amount of sodium the patient will receive over the whole treatment schedule. Give your answer in milligrams to the nearest whole number.

349 As part of a clinical trial a subject has been commenced on a novel anti-epileptic drug and tests are monitoring the drug levels in the body as well as rate of excretion. The initial drug blood levels are 1280 micrograms/mL and 60 hours later, they have fallen to 20 micrograms/mL. Assuming that no more of the drug is administered and that the new drug excretion obeys first order kinetics, calculate the half-life of the drug. Give your answer in hours.

350 You are working as a GP practice pharmacist and are reviewing patents who have been prescribed doxazosin oral solution to potentially change them to tablets that can be crushed as a cost saving exercise for the practice. Currently there are 19 patients who are prescribed doxazosin oral solution 4mg/5mL at a dose of 4 milligrams daily. If 150 mL of doxazosin 4mg/5mL costs £50.60 and 28 doxazosin 4mg tablets cost £0.92, calculate the amount the practice will save over 90 days if all patients were switched to tablets. Give your answer to the nearest £10.

351 A patient has been commenced on a course of chlormethiazole to manage alcohol withdrawal. The dose prescribed is as follows:
- 4 capsules TDS on day 1
- 4 capsules BD on day 2
- 3 capsules BD on day 3
- 2 capsules BD on days 4,5 and 6
- 1 capsule BD on days 7 & 8
- 1 capsule on day 9 and then stop.

Due to a recent illness, the patient can no longer swallow capsules and so the formulation has been changed to a solution for ease of ingestion. Chlormethiazole is available as a 31.54 mg/mL oral solution where 157.7mg is equivalent to a single 192mg capsule. Calculate how much solution, in millilitres, is needed to cover the 9 days of treatment for this patient.

352 A patient weighing 70kg has been admitted to hospital following a liver transplant and has been prescribed tacrolimus at a dose of 50micrograms/kg delivered via an infusion over 24 hours to supress transplant rejection. Tacrolimus is available as a 0.001% w/v infusion. What infusion rate does the patient need to receive in mL per hour? Give your answer to 2 decimal places.

353 You have a 2000mL infusion bag containing glucose 20%. You discard 250mL of the infusion bag and replace with 500ml of glucose 60%. What is the final concentration (% w/v) of the infusion bag? Give your answer to 2 decimal places.

354 A patient has been admitted to the respiratory ward and is having their theophylline levels measured as they are showing signs of toxicity. The patient is currently taking a dose of theophylline MR tablets 300mg BD. Theophylline has a half-life of 8 hours and is excreted following first order kinetics. If the patients' current blood plasma levels of theophylline are 400 micrograms per litre, how long will it take for concentration levels to reach 25 micrograms per litre assuming the patient takes no further doses?

355 A patient weighing 43kg requires treatment to manage iron deficiency anaemia. They have been prescribed a dose of 3mg/kg of ferrous iron daily, orally for 56 days before a review is needed. If ferrous sulfate 200mg is equivalent to 65mg of ferrous iron, calculate how many ferrous sulfate 200mg tablets are needed to cover the treatment period before review.

356 A patient has commenced a reducing dose of prednisolone following a COPD exacerbation. The current treatment schedule is 45mg for seven days and then reduce by 5mg every seven days until taking 5mg daily for 28 days and then stop. How many full packets of 28 prednisolone 5mg tablets are needed to cover the entire course of treatment?

357 You have been asked to calculate the correct dose of lidocaine for a patient to manage ventricular arrhythmia following a myocardial infarction. The patient weighs 61 kg and has been prescribed a dose of 4mg/kg using 0.5% lidocaine w/v solution to be administered as a single dose. How many mL of lidocaine 0.5% w/v solution for injection needs to be administered? Give your answer to 1 decimal place.

358 A 52-year-old patient weighing 71kg has been prescribed Oramorph® concentrate oral solution 100mg/5mL. The prescribed dose is 60mg when required up to a maximum of four times a day for breakthrough pain as they are currently on morphine sulfate MR tablets 60mg BD. What is the volume in mL required for each dose for breakthrough pain.

359 A patient has been prescribed 500mg amoxicillin capsules with directions to take one capsule three times a day for seven days. Calculate, in grams, the total weight of amoxicillin taken by the patient by the end of the course. Give your answer to 1 decimal place.

360 A 63-year-old patient has been prescribed co-codamol 30/500mg effervescent tablets. The dose the patient takes is two tablets TDS. Each tablet contains 388mg of sodium. The recommended daily allowance of salt for an adult is 6 g (equivalent to 2.4 g sodium) per day. What percentage of this patient's recommended daily sodium allowance is contained in their total daily dose of co-codamol 30/500mg effervescent tablets?

361 A 62-year-old male patient who weighs 63Kg, has been admitted to your ward. Their latest serum creatinine level is 250micromol/L. They have been prescribed a new medication, drug X which is mostly excreted through the kidneys. Due to the renal excretion, the dose must be adjusted depending on the patient's renal function calculated using the Cockcroft-Gault formula and applied as follows:

Creatinine Clearance (mL/min)	Dosage
< 10	10mg/kg every 12 hours
10 - 20	15mg/kg every 12 hours
21 - 35	20mg/kg every 8 hours
35 - 50	25mg/kg every 8 hours
> 50	27.5mg/kg every 8 hours

Cockcroft-Gault equation:

Estimated creatinine clearance in mL/min = (140 − age (years)) × weight (kg) × constant ÷ serum creatinine (micromol/L)

Constant = 1.23 for men, 1.04 for women

What dose of Drug X would you recommend to be taken over a 24 hour period? Give your answer in grams to 2 decimal places.

362 A 32-year-old patient weighing 71kg requires treatment with a 1.2g stat dose of benzylpenicillin for suspected meningococcal disease. Benzylpenicillin is available as vials containing powder for reconstitution. A single vial contains 600mg. The displacement volume of a 600mg vial is 0.4mL. It is recommended that the vial is reconstituted with water for

injections to a final concentration of 30mg/mL. How many milliliters of water for injection is needed to reconstitute each vial of benzylpenicillin to the concentration requested? Give your answer to one decimal place.

363 A 61-year-old man is admitted to your ward for treatment of herpes simplex infection with aciclovir at a dose of 7.5mg/kg. The patient weighs 46kg and has a serum creatinine of 120micromoles/L. You have the following information about the use of aciclovir:

Dosage adjustments in adults and adolescents:

Creatinine Clearance	Dosage
25 to 50 ml/min	The recommended dose (5 - 10mg/kg body weight) should be given every 8 hours.
10 to 25 ml/min	The recommended dose (5 - 10mg/kg body weight) should be given every 12 hours
0 (anuric) to 10 ml/min	In patients receiving continuous ambulatory peritoneal dialysis (CAPD) the dose recommended above (5 - 10 mg/kg body weight) should be halved and administered every 24 hours. In patients receiving haemodialysis the dose recommended above (5 - 10mg/kg body weight) should be halved and administered every 24 hours and after dialysis.

Cockcroft-Gault equation:

Estimated creatinine clearance in mL/min = (140 − age (years)) × weight (kg) × constant serum creatinine (micromol/L)

Constant = 1.23 for men, 1.04 for women

What is the recommended number of hours between doses of aciclovir for this patient?

364 You are working in a pharmaceutical laboratory and have a stock solution of a new drug with a concentration of 63% w/v. The drug is used as a mouthwash at a concentration of 0.475% w/v. You are requested to prepare 75mL of a solution of intermediate strength, such that those using the mouthwash will dilute this solution 1 in 10 to get the correct concentration immediately before use. What would be the concentration of the intermediate solution? Give you answer 2 decimal places.

365 A patient has congestive heart failure and is to receive digoxin. They weigh 69kg and have an estimated creatinine clearance of 28mL/minute. Using the information provided, calculate the patient's digoxin clearance. Give your answer to the nearest whole number.

For patients without heart failure:
Digoxin clearance (mL/minute)
= (0.8 × weight in kg) + creatinine clearance (mL/minute)

For patients with congestive heart failure:
Digoxin clearance (mL/minute)
= (0.33 × weight in kg) + (0.9 × creatinine clearance mL/minute)

366 A 38-year-old woman is receiving her first infusion of etoposide following a recent diagnosis of ovarian cancer. Working as an oncology pharmacist you are to clinically screen the etoposide infusion prescription. The patient's most recent measured creatinine clearance was 37mL/min. She weighs 62kg and is 156cm tall. The medical team would like her to receive the same dose for five consecutive days, using the upper limit of the dosing range. The formula for body surface area has been provided here:

$$BSA = \sqrt{\frac{(height\ (cm) \times weight\ (kg))}{3600}}$$

Use the information about posology and method of administration (section 4.2) in the link below to answer the following question: *https://www.medicines.org.uk/emc/product/9070/smpc*
How many milligrams of etoposide would the patient receive on day 1 of chemotherapy? Give your answer to the nearest whole number.

367 A 32-year-old patient requires treatment with ceftazidime to treat febrile neutropenia. Using the extract provided, calculate the infusion rate to be

set in mL/min if the infusion is administered over 30 minutes. Give your answer to 1 decimal place.
Extract: *https://bnf.nice.org.uk/drugs/ceftazidime/#indications-and-dose*

368 A 75-year-old female has been prescribed a trial drug to treat Hodgkin lymphoma. She has been prescribed a dose of 10mg/m2 daily for 3 days. The patient weighs 55kg and is 1.8m tall. The trial drug is available as 5mg vials. How many vials are needed to complete the full course?

$$BSA = \sqrt{\frac{(\text{height (cm)} \times \text{weight (kg)})}{3600}}$$

369 A 73-year-old female patient has been diagnosed with atrial fibrillation. The cardiologist has prescribed an intravenous infusion of digoxin. You have been asked by a doctor to calculate a suitable loading dose for digoxin for the patient. The patient weighs 68kg. The target digoxin concentration is 80microgram/L. Using the provided formulae, calculate a suitable loading dose in milligrams for this patient. Give your answer to 1 decimal place.

$$\begin{aligned}
\text{loading dose (mcg)} &= (VD \times \text{concentration}) \div (F \times S) \\
\text{Volume of distribution (VD)} &= 0.15 \text{L/kg} \\
\text{Bioavailability (F)} &= 1 \\
\text{Salt factor (S)} &= 0.88
\end{aligned}$$

370 A 17-year-old child has an infected wound. The child has been prescribed potassium permanganate solution 1 in 4000. This product is prepared from a stock solution of 30 times this strength. How much potassium permanganate stock solution will be needed if the child uses 150 mL of the diluted solution twice a day for 14 days? Give your answer to 2 decimal places in litres.

371 You are working in the aseptic unit of a hospital. You have been requested to supply 500mL of a solution of intermediate strength such that the patient will dilute this solution 1 in 5 times to get the correct concentration immediately before use. You have a stock solution at 30% concentration. The solution is used at a concentration of 4% w/v. How many millilitres of diluent are needed to make 500mL of the intermediate solution? Give your answer to 1 decimal place.

372 You have been asked to prepare 30 suppositories with each containing 50mg of magnesium sulphate in theobroma oil base. Each suppository will be made to a 200mg mould. You are required to make a surplus of 20% to account for any loss during production. Given that the displacement value of magnesium sulphate in theobroma oil base is 1.5, how much base will be required?

373 You are working on a hospital ward and have been asked for advice by a nurse on how to prepare sodium valproate injection for administration. The displacement volume of sodium valproate is 0.6 mL/600 mg. Calculate the volume of solvent (water for injection) required to be added to a vial containing 300 mg sodium valproate to produce a solution with a concentration of 100mg/mL. Give your answer to one decimal place.

374 You are working for the Integrated Care Boards (ICB) and are involved in cost-saving projects. You are reviewing the cost saving if patients are switched from branded apixaban to generic. Costs are shown below:

Drug	Cost	Dose
Apixaban 5mg (generic)	£15.73/60 tabs	1 tablet BD
Eliquis 5mg (brand)	£43.12/60 tabs	1 tablet BD

You have reviewed 30 patients who are prescribed branded apixaban and of those patients, 90% can be switched to generic. The practice has a repeat prescribing policy of 30 days treatment of prescription. What is the total saving for 3 repeats assuming all the eligible patients switch to the generic form? Give your answer to the nearest £10.

375 You are taking part in the clinical research of a trial drug. 7.5% of patients receiving a new cholesterol medication known as Drug X experienced unacceptable adverse effects compared to only 2.5% using standard treatment. Calculate the number needed to harm for patients receiving the new drug.

Number Needed to Harm (NNH) = 100/ARI (Absolute Risk Increase)
ARI = EER (Experiment Event Rate %) − CER (Control Event Rate %)

376 You are a practice pharmacist synchronising a patient's repeat medication so that all their medication can be ordered once a month, instead of several times a month.

	Strength	Dose	Quantity left
Amlodipine	10 mg	Take ONE daily	27
Bisoprolol	3.75 mg	Take ONE twice a day	18
Colecalciferol	1000 units	Take ONE in the morning	18
Glimepiride	3 mg	Take ONE daily	23
Metformin	500 mg	Take TWO twice a day	28
Lisinopril	10 mg	Take ONE daily	5
Omeprazole	20 mg	Take ONE daily	27

How many additional metformin 500mg tablets should be prescribed to synchronise the patient's medications?

377 A patient has been admitted to hospital due to an exacerbation of ulcerative colitis. Due to the risk of adrenal suppression, the patient has been discharged on a reducing dose of prednisolone. The patient has been prescribed 40mg daily with instructions to reduce by 5mg every 3 days until taking 5mg and then to continue this dose for 7 days before stopping. How many 5mg tablets would the patient need to be discharged with?

378 A 73-year-old male patient has been prescribed Maxidex® (dexamethasone) eye drops for his right eye following cataract surgery. The patient has been instructed to 'instil ONE drop into the affected eye four times a day starting one day prior to surgery, continue on the day of the surgery and for the first two weeks' of the postoperative period. Maxidex® 0.1% w/v, eye drops, suspension: 20 drops is equivalent to 1mL. Available in 5mL bottle. Calculate the volume in millilitres that will remain in the bottle after following the prescriber's instruction (assuming all drops were given)? Give your answer to 1 decimal place.

379 A child has been prescribed lansoprazole 15mg dispersible tablets. The parent has been advised to dissolve one 15mg tablet in 10mL of water before administering the required dose. How many millilitres of the resulting solution should be given to the child to provide a 6mg daily dose?

380 You receive the following prescription for a 14-year-old child weighing 40kg for the management of Kawasaki disease. How long will it take to complete the whole infusion if it was infused at the prescribed rate?

Today's date	Immunoglobulin 16% 0.8g/kg	0.8mL/kg/hr for 30 mins then	Doctor D.
		1.2mL/kg/hr for 40 mins then	
		1.8mL/kg/hr for 50 mins then	
		3mL/kg/hr for the remainder of the infusion	

381 A 10-year-old child weighing 38kg has been prescribed levetiracetam intravenous infusion for the management of epilepsy. The child has been prescribed a dose of 50mg/kg/day in two divided doses. Levetiracetam is available as 500mg/5mL intravenous infusion and should be administered over 20 minutes, as per trust guidelines. What rate should the infusion be set at per dose in mL/min? Give your answer to 2 decimal places.

382 A 55-year-old male has bowel impaction and has been advised to take 8 sachets of Laxido® a day for the next 5 days. The atomic mass of sodium is 23 and the atomic mass of chloride is 35.5. Each sachet contains 12mmol of sodium chloride. The recommended daily intake of sodium chloride is 6g. What percentage of the sodium chloride recommended daily allowance will the patient receive from the sachets if taken as directed? Give your answer to 1 decimal place.

383 A 68-year-old male has been found to have severe hypokalaemia. His latest serum potassium level was 2.4mmol/L (normal range: 4.5-5.5 mmol/L). He has since been prescribed 1.5L of 40mmol potassium chloride (KCl) solution in 500mL of sodium chloride 0.9% pre-filled infusion bags.

Relative Molecular Mass (RMM) of KCl is 74.5

Calculate the amount potassium chloride in grams the patient will receive upon completing the whole infusion? Give your answer to 1 decimal place.

384 A 65-year-old male weighs 80kg and has been prescribed VTE prophylaxis using tinzaparin. You are clinically checking if the dose of tinzaparin is appropriate; to do this you need to calculate the patient's renal function. His latest serum creatinine level was 98micromol/L. Calculate the creatinine clearance (mL/min) using the Cockcroft-Gault formula provided. Give your answer to the nearest whole number.

Cockcroft-Gault equation:

Estimated creatinine clearance in mL/min = (140 − age (years)) × weight (kg) × constant serum creatinine (micromol/L)

Constant = 1.23 for men, 1.04 for women

385 A 58-year-old man weighing 88kg is 5 foot 6 inches (2.81 m2) tall. The patient has a complicated skin infection and has been prescribed IV vancomycin* as advised by microbiology. An initial loading dose was administered, and you have been asked to calculate the patient's renal function*. His serum creatinine is 136micromol/litre.
*When using vancomycin the renal function should be calculated using the patients ideal body weight (IBW) if the BMI is >30.

IBW Male (kg) = 50 + (2.3 × number of inches above 5 ft in height)
IBW Female (kg) = 45.5 (2.3 × number of inches above 5 ft in height)

Calculate the renal function of the patient. Give your answer to 1 decimal place.

Cockcroft-Gault equation:

Estimated creatinine clearance in mL/min = (140 − age (years)) × weight (kg) × constant serum creatinine (micromol/L)

Constant = 1.23 for men, 1.04 for women

386 A 23-year-old female is taking Drug X to manage an autoimmune disease. According to the SPC the half-life of Drug X is 4 hours. The initial plasma level of the drug after a single dose was 4,480mg/L. The plasma level is now 2,187.5 microgram/L. How many minutes have passed since the initial dose?

387 A 57-year-old female has been administered a trial drug. The half-life of the drug is 3 hours. The initial plasma level of the drug after a single dose was 1,000mg/L. What will the drug plasma level be at 18 hours? Give your answer to 1 decimal place in mg/L.

388 You are a hospital pharmacist working on a surgical ward. A patient has undergone bariatric surgery, the trust guideline advises for the patient to be switched to a liquid formulation where possible for the first 6 weeks post operation. You have been asked for advice by a junior doctor on switching a patient's phenytoin tablets to liquid. The patient is currently prescribed phenytoin 200mg tablets three times a day. Phenytoin suspension* is available as 30mg/5mL in a 500mL bottle. The syringe available is graduated at 0.5mL intervals. Calculate the volume of phenytoin suspension required per dose in millilitres? Give your answer to 1 decimal place.
*Phenytoin 100mg tablets – are equivalent to 92mg oral suspension

389 You are pharmacist working on a stroke ward. A patient has developed difficulty swallowing following a stroke. You have been asked to convert the patient's digoxin tablets* to a liquid preparation for ease of swallowing before discharge. The patient was originally taking digoxin 250 microgram tablets once daily. Calculate the number of bottles of digoxin needed for a 14-day supply on discharge.
*Digoxin: 62.5microgram tablet equivalent to 50microgram (in 1mL) elixir. Each bottle contains 60mL.

390 You have in stock a 450mL glucose 50% (w/v) solution. You receive a prescription to produce a new solution by removing 250mL of the stock solution and replacing it with 200mL of glucose 20% (w/v) solution. What is the percentage concentration of the new solution in %w/v?

391 A drug is available in a vial containing 1g powder for solution for injection. 250mg of powder for solution for injection has a displacement volume of 0.5mL and contains 30mg of the drug. Each vial must be diluted with 8mL of water for injection prior to administration. What is the concentration of the drug in mg/mL in the reconstituted vial?

Case based discussion questions

Questions 392-400 are suggested areas of discussion/revision.

392 A 28-year-old patient visits the community pharmacy and would like to discuss travel advice with you. She is planning on travelling to South America for 3 months. What will you discuss with the patient?

393 A 37-year-old patient (Mr GC) visits the community pharmacy and would like to discuss nicotine replacement therapy. Which is the most appropriate nicotine product to supply to the patient?

394 Ms FY, a 22-year-old patient visits the community pharmacy and is requesting emergency hormonal contraception. Unprotected sexual intercourse took place 2 days ago. How do you manage the patient?

395 Mr GL (62 years) is initiated on warfarin for atrial fibrillation prophylaxis. What counselling does he require?

396 A 5-year-old patient is diagnosed with headlice. How do you manage the patient?

397 You are discussing diseases with the healthcare assistant. She informs you that she has recently read about the term 'notifiable diseases'. What does this term mean and how will it be relevant to your practice?

398 A colleague has been sharing patient identifiable data/information on social media. You are aware it may have happened unintentionally. How do you manage the situation?

399 Part I. A 21-year-old patient would like to purchase over the counter contraception? What is available OTC and how can you safely supply?

399 Part II. A 55-year-old female patient would like to purchase over the counter HRT medication? Is anything available?

400 You are the responsible pharmacist in a community pharmacy. What does this responsibility mean? What are your legal obligations during this role? Are you able to have a break?

High weighted answers

1 **A – Carbamazepine**
Antiepileptic hypersensitivity syndrome is a rare but potentially fatal syndrome associated with some antiepileptic drugs (carbamazepine, lacosamide, lamotrigine, oxcarbazepine, phenobarbital, phenytoin, primidone, and rufinamide); rarely cross-sensitivity occurs between some of these antiepileptic drugs. The symptoms usually start between 1 and 8 weeks of exposure; fever, rash, and lymphadenopathy are most commonly seen. Other systemic signs include liver dysfunction, haematological, renal, and pulmonary abnormalities, vasculitis, and multi-organ failure. If signs or symptoms of hypersensitivity syndrome occur, the drug should be withdrawn immediately, the patient must not be re-exposed, and expert advice should be sought.
https://bnf.nice.org.uk/drugs/carbamazepine/#patient-and-carer-advice

2 **C – 6 months**
The DVLA recommends that patients should not drive during medication changes or withdrawal of antiepileptic drugs, and for 6 months after their last dose. If a seizure occurs due to a prescribed change or withdrawal of epilepsy treatment, the patient will have their driving license revoked for 1 year; relicensing may be considered earlier if treatment has been reinstated for 6 months and no further seizures have occurred.
https://www.gov.uk/epilepsy-and-driving

3 **E – Tramadol**
Tramadol can lower seizure threshold. In BNF monograph epileptiform seizure is listed as a side effect of tramadol. From social history, the patient appears to consume alcohol in excess. The seizure threshold is raised by alcohol drinking and declines on cessation of drinking. As a result, during withdrawal from alcohol, usually 6-48 hours after the cessation of

drinking, seizures may occur. As such, it is important in this case to also ascertain the patient's recent alcohol intake.
https://bnf.nice.org.uk/drugs/tramadol-hydrochloride/#side-effects

4   **B – Gradually reduce the dose of rotigotine**
Impulse control disorders can develop in a person with Parkinson's disease who is on any dopaminergic therapy at any stage in the disease course. Being on dopamine agonist therapy, having a history of previous impulsive behaviours and alcohol consumption and/or smoking are associated with an increased risk of developing impulse control disorders. When managing impulse control disorders, modify dopaminergic therapy by first gradually reducing any dopamine agonist. Monitor whether the impulse control disorder improves and whether the person has any symptoms of dopamine agonist withdrawal. Offer specialist cognitive behavioural therapy targeted at impulse control disorders if modifying dopaminergic therapy is not effective.
https://bnf.nice.org.uk/drugs/rotigotine/#indications-and-dose

5   **A – Discontinue the antipsychotic treatment**
The symptoms are suggestive of neuroleptic malignant syndrome (NMS) which is a rare but potentially fatal side-effect of all antipsychotic drugs. NMS are characterised by hyperthermia, fluctuating level of consciousness, muscle rigidity, and autonomic dysfunction with fever, tachycardia, labile blood pressure, and sweating. Expert sources advise discontinuation of the antipsychotic drug is essential for at least 5 days, preferably longer. The signs and symptoms of neuroleptic malignant syndrome should be allowed to resolve completely. Bromocriptine and dantrolene have been used for treatment.
https://cks.nice.org.uk/topics/psychosis-schizophrenia/prescribing-information/adverse-effects/

6   **F – Switch the antipsychotic treatment to aripiprazole**
Most antipsychotic drugs, both first- and second-generation, increase prolactin concentration to some extent because dopamine inhibits prolactin release. The clinical symptoms of hyperprolactinaemia include sexual dysfunction, reduced bone mineral density, menstrual disturbances, breast enlargement, galactorrhoea, and a possible increased

risk of breast cancer. Risperidone, amisulpride, sulpiride, and first-generation antipsychotics (such as trifluoperazine) are most likely to cause symptomatic hyperprolactinaemia. Olanzapine is not suitable in this case due to its metabolic side effects – the patient has a background of diabetes and obesity. Aripiprazole reduces prolactin concentration in a dose-dependent manner because it is a dopamine-receptor partial agonist.
https://bnf.nice.org.uk/drugs/aripiprazole/

7   **C – Start hyoscine hydrobromide up to 300microgram three times a day**
Hypersalivation associated with clozapine therapy can be treated with hyoscine hydrobromide (unlicensed indication), provided that the patient is not at particular risk from the additive antimuscarinic side-effects of hyoscine and clozapine.
https://bnf.nice.org.uk/drugs/hyoscine-hydrobromide/#indications-and-dose

8   **A – Discontinue the antipsychotic treatment**
The symptoms are tardive dyskinesia, which can develop on long-term or high-dose antipsychotic therapy, or even after discontinuation; in some patients it can be irreversible. Tardive dyskinesia is characterised by abnormal involuntary movements of lips, tongue, face, and jaw. Tardive dyskinesia is the most serious manifestation of late-onset extrapyramidal symptoms for which there is no satisfactory treatment; it occurs more commonly in elderly females. Some manufacturers suggest that drug withdrawal at the earliest signs of tardive dyskinesia (fine vermicular movements of the tongue) may halt its full development. Tardive dyskinesia is not improved by procyclidine and may be made worse.
https://cks.nice.org.uk/topics/psychosis-schizophrenia/prescribing-information/adverse-effects/

9   **D – Sertraline**
SSRIs are the agents of choice in CHD. They are generally safe and well tolerated in patients with CHD when appropriate precautions are taken. NICE recommends for people with depression who also have a chronic physical health problem to consider using citalopram and sertraline are first line as these have a lower propensity for interactions. Sertraline is safe post MI and considered the drug of choice. Tricyclic antidepressants

are known to be cardiotoxic. Therefore, TCAs are best avoided in patients with CHD and are contraindicated in patients who have had a recent MI. NICE advises that tricyclic antidepressants, except for lofepramine, are associated with the greatest risk in overdose. Mirtazapine is a suitable alternative in cardiac disease if SSRIs cannot be used but it should be used with caution. There is evidence of safety post MI. Venlafaxine is contraindicated in patients with an identified high risk of a serious cardiac ventricular arrhythmia or with uncontrolled hypertension. It should be used with caution in established cardiac disease that may increase the risk of ventricular arrhythmias (e.g. recent myocardial infarction). Venlafaxine is associated with a greater risk of death from overdose compared with other equally effective antidepressants.
https://www.sps.nhs.uk/articles/choosing-an-antidepressant-for-people-with-coronary-heart-disease/#:~:text=SSRIs%20 are%20the%20preferred%20antidepressants%20in%20CHD.%20 Sertraline%2C,Mirtazapine%20is%20also%20a%20preferred%20 antidepressant%20in%20CHD.

10   **C – Citalopram, methadone and ondansetron.**
QTc is prolonged if >440ms in men or >470ms in women. Citalopram, methadone and ondansetron can prolong QTc interval. The manufacturer advises that the use of two or more drugs that are associated with QTc prolongation should be avoided where possible. Print versions of the BNF contain a table with a list of drugs that prolong the QT interval.
BNF (Print) Appendix 1, Interactions

11   **A – Amlodipine**
The first line antihypertensive for this patient, according to the NICE guidance, is ramipril. However, as the patient is also taking lithium, which is a narrow therapeutic index drug, interactions with other drugs needs to be considered. The most commonly encountered interactions are with:
- Diuretics — thiazide diuretics can cause a rapid increase in serum lithium levels (7–10 days) by reducing clearance of lithium. The increase in lithium levels varies from 25–400% Loop diuretics also cause lithium retention but are less likely to result in lithium toxicity.
- ACE inhibitors/angiotensin-II receptor antagonists decrease the excretion of lithium. They can also precipitate renal failure. If these

two drugs are prescribed together, extra care is required in monitoring both serum creatinine and lithium levels.

As such, amlodipine is the most appropriate option. Doxazosin does not have clinically significant interaction with lithium but it is 4th line antihypertensive according to the NICE guideline so should not be initiated at this point.
https://www.nice.org.uk/guidance/ng136

12   **E – Thyroid function test**
Presenting symptoms are indicative of hypothyroidism. There is a small risk that people taking lithium at therapeutic doses may develop clinical goitre, hypothyroidism, or both; the risk appears to be greatest in the first 2 years of treatment. Although this may occur, it should not be a reason for stopping lithium treatment. Levothyroxine replacement is usually indicated. Thyroxine function tests usually return to normal when lithium is discontinued.
https://www.sps.nhs.uk/monitorings/lithium-monitoring/

13   **A – One week after dose change, at 12 hours after dose**
Lithium levels are normally measured one week after starting treatment, one week after every dose change, and weekly until the levels are stable. Once levels are stable, levels are usually measured every 3 months. Lithium levels should be measured 12 hours post-dose.
https://bnf.nice.org.uk/drugs/lithium-carbonate/#monitoring-requirements

14   **G – ORBIT**
Although both HAS-BLED and ORBIT scores are recognised tool to assess bleeding risk with anticoagulation, the current NICE guidelines for diagnosis and management of atrial fibrillation (updated 2021) recommends the use of ORBIT score. This is because evidence suggested that ORBIT was more accurate than HAS-BLED at predicting absolute risk of major bleeding, both for people using vitamin K antagonists and those using direct-acting oral anticoagulant. ORBIT was also better at predicting absolute risk of intracranial haemorrhage.

   Additional information: It is important to note that bleeding risk tool should not be used to provide a cut off for determining who should

have anticoagulation. Instead, the tool should be used to provide accurate knowledge of absolute bleeding risk, which can support discussions between the person and their healthcare professional about bleeding risk modification and appropriate levels of vigilance.
https://www.nice.org.uk/guidance/ng196 AND *https://www.mdcalc.com/calc/10227/orbit-bleeding-risk-score-atrial-fibrillation* AND *https://www.mdcalc.com/calc/807/has-bled-score-major-bleeding-risk*

15 **B – GRACE**
In patients who have been diagnosed with NSTEMI or unstable angina, GRACE score is the formal risk assessment tool to assess and categorise risk of future adverse cardiovascular events. This is important for determining early management strategies as it allows the benefits of treatment to be balanced against the risks of treatment-related adverse events. Failure to categorise future risk can lead to people being given inappropriate treatment.
https://www.mdcalc.com/calc/1099/grace-acs-risk-mortality-calculator

16 **F – NYHA**
Heart failure can be classified in terms of ejection fraction, time course of heart failure and symptomatic severity. The New York Heart Association (NYHA) is the functional classification of heart failure based on severity of symptoms and limitation of physical activity.
https://cks.nice.org.uk/topics/heart-failure-chronic/
https://cks.nice.org.uk/topics/heart-failure-chronic/background-information/definition/

17 **E – No disease classification or risk scoring system exists**
The patient in this scenario has established coronary artery disease. As such, it is inappropriate to use a primary prevention risk took, such as QRISK3, to assess his risk of developing future cardiovascular event.
https://www.qrisk.org/

18 **F – Nicorandil**
Nicorandil can cause serious skin, mucosal, and eye ulceration; including gastrointestinal ulcers, which may progress to perforation, haemorrhage, fistula or abscess. Stop treatment if ulceration occurs and consider an alternative.
https://bnf.nice.org.uk/drugs/nicorandil/

19 **C – Dapagliflozin**
Sodium-glucose co-transporter 2 (SGLT-2) inhibitors (canagliflozin, dapagliflozin or empagliflozin) are associated with risk of diabetic ketoacidosis. Treatment with a SGLT-2 inhibitor should be withheld in patients who are hospitalised for major surgery or acute serious illnesses, treatment may be restarted once the patient's condition has stabilised.
https://bnf.nice.org.uk/treatment-summaries/type-2-diabetes/

20 **E – Dalteparin sodium 15,000 units S/C OD**
Section 4.2 of Fragmin SPC (use month 2-6 Table as patient has been on Fragmin for 5 weeks): 83-98kg dose is 15,000 units OD. There is no renal impairment so there is no need for Anti-Xa level monitoring.

21 **B – Dalteparin sodium 5,000 units S/C OD**
Section 4.2 of Fragmin SPC - Prophylaxis of venous thromboembolism in medical patients: The recommended dose of dalteparin sodium is 5,000 IU once daily. Note local hospital guidelines may suggest a reduced dalteparin dose in patients <45kg/50kg – this is evidence-based due to risk of accumulation of the drug in low BW patients. However, as the question asks you to use the SPC, the licensed dose for dalteparin in thromboprophylaxis as per the SPC is 5000units OD (regardless of weight).

22 **B – Aspirin 75mg OD and Dipyridamole M/R 200mg BD**
The standard antiplatelet therapy following a TIA is clopidogrel 75 mg OD. Aspirin 75mg OD with modified-release dipyridamole 200mg BD may be used if clopidogrel cannot be tolerated.
   Modified-release dipyridamole 200mg BD may be used if both clopidogrel and aspirin are contraindicated or cannot be tolerated. Aspirin 75mg OD may be used if both clopidogrel and modified-release dipyridamole are contraindicated or cannot be tolerated. Dual therapy with aspirin plus clopidogrel (for up to 90 days) or aspirin plus ticagrelor (for 30 days) may be initiated in secondary care for some people (for example people at high risk of TIA, or those with intracranial stenosis) followed by antiplatelet monotherapy.

23 **D – Doxorubicin**
Anthracycline chemotherapy (doxorubicin, daunorubicin, epirubicin

and idarubicin) causes dose-related cardiomyocyte injury and death, leading to left ventricular dysfunction. Clinical heart failure may ensue in up to 5% of high-risk patients. Echocardiogram is performed at the start of treatment to establish baseline, and routine monitoring of left ventricular function is performed every 3 months during treatment. The risk of cardiotoxicity increases with cumulative doses.
https://bnf.nice.org.uk/drugs/doxorubicin-hydrochloride-specialist-drug/#indications-and-dose

24   **E – Verapamil**
The patient's blood pressure is 94/56 mmHg and his heart rate is 56bpm, so he is both hypotensive and bradycardic. Verapamil is a rate-limiting CCB so affects both BP and pulse. Stopping ramipril is also appropriate (as will help with hypotension) however the question asks for the most important drug to be stopped.
https://bnf.nice.org.uk/drugs/verapamil-hydrochloride/#indications-and-dose

25   **D – Rivaroxaban**
This is a recognised interaction. Rifampicin is a CYP450 inducer so it is predicted to decrease the exposure to Rivaroxaban. Manufacturer advises avoid. Patient should be switched to warfarin during the duration of antibiotics and for 4-6 weeks after.
https://bnf.nice.org.uk/drugs/rivaroxaban/ AND https://www.medicines.org.uk/emc/product/15707/smpc

26   **B – 20mg**
The maximum recommended dose for simvastatin in conjunction with amlodipine or diltiazem is now 20 mg/day as per MHRA guidance.
https://www.gov.uk/drug-safety-update/simvastatin-dose-limitations-with-concomitant-amlodipine-or-diltiazem

27   **D – all of the above**
Following an acute coronary syndrome such as an NSTEMI, patients must be started on a range of medications to prevent a secondary cardiovascular event. These include an angiotensin-converting enzyme (ACE) inhibitor, a beta blocker, dual antiplatelet therapy and a statin.
See BNF treatment summaries - Acute coronary syndromes.

28 **B – Labetalol**
First line treatment of hypertension in pregnancy is labetalol. ACE inhibitors, ARBs, thiazide or thiazide like diuretics should be avoided. See NICE guidelines – Hypertension in pregnancy.
https://www.nice.org.uk/guidance/ng133

29 **D – Enalapril**
Post birth, the first line of treatment is enalapril. In females of black African or African Caribbean family origin, nifedipine or amlodipine should be considered first line. See NICE guidelines – Hypertension in pregnancy
https://www.nice.org.uk/guidance/ng133

30 **E – Verapamil**
Verapamil can precipitate heart failure, exacerbate conduction disorders, and cause hypotension at high doses and should not be used with beta-blockers. See BNF treatment summaries – Calcium-channel blockers.
https://bnf.nice.org.uk/treatment-summaries/calcium-channel-blockers/

31 **B – Fluvastatin 80mg**
See BNF treatment summaries – Dyslipidaemias.
https://bnf.nice.org.uk/treatment-summaries/dyslipidaemias/

32 **C – For plasma-drug concentration, blood should be taken at least 4 hrs after a dose**
Plasma-drug concentration should be taken at least 6 hrs after a dose. See BNF Drug monograph for digoxin.
https://bnf.nice.org.uk/drugs/digoxin/

33 **F – Flucloxacillin**
See BNF treatment summaries - diabetic foot infections, antibacterial therapy.
https://bnf.nice.org.uk/treatment-summaries/diabetic-foot-infections-antibacterial-therapy/

34 **D – Co-amoxiclav**
See BNF treatment summaries – gastrointestinal system infections, antibacterial therapy.
https://bnf.nice.org.uk/treatment-summaries/gastro-intestinal-system-infections-antibacterial-therapy/

35 **C – Clarithromycin**
    See BNF treatment summaries – ear infections, antibacterial therapy.
    https://bnf.nice.org.uk/treatment-summaries/ear-infections-antibacterial-therapy/

36 **H – Metronidazole**
    See BNF treatment summaries – genital system infections, antibacterial therapy.
    https://bnf.nice.org.uk/treatment-summaries/genital-system-infections-antibacterial-therapy/

37 **D – Co-amoxiclav**
    See BNF treatment summaries – skin infections, antibacterial therapy.
    https://bnf.nice.org.uk/treatment-summaries/skin-infections-antibacterial-therapy/

38 **D – Co-amoxiclav**
    See BNF treatment summaries – respiratory system infections, antibacterial therapy.
    https://bnf.nice.org.uk/treatment-summaries/respiratory-system-infections-antibacterial-therapy/

39 **C – Doxycycline**
    Doxycycline can cause the skin to be more sensitive to sunlight than it is normally. Exposure to sunlight, even for short periods of time, may cause skin rash, itching, redness or other discoloration of the skin, or a severe sunburn.
    https://bnf.nice.org.uk/drugs/doxycycline/#patient-and-carer-advice

40 **D – Ceftriaxone**
    Ceftriaxone and cefotaxime can cross the blood-brain barrier making it a suitable antibiotic for treating infections of the central nervous system.
    https://www.medicines.org.uk/emc/product/2407/smpc#gref

41 **B – Gentamicin can be diluted with 0.9% sodium chloride or 10% glucose solution**
    Special precautions for disposable and other handling - Gentamicin can be diluted with 0.9% sodium chloride or 5% glucose solution.
    https://www.medicines.org.uk/emc/product/2407/smpc#gref (see section 6.3)

42 D – Metronidazole
Alcohol should be avoided until 48 hours after stopping metronidazole. Drinking alcohol with metronidazole can cause side effects such as flushing of the face, vomiting and stomach pains.
https://bnf.nice.org.uk/interactions/metronidazole/

43 D – Simvastatin
Risk factors for muscle toxicity, including myopathy or rhabdomyolysis are cautioned for all statins.
https://bnf.nice.org.uk/drugs/simvastatin/

44 E – Sertraline
In patients with unstable angina or who have had a recent myocardial infarction, sertraline has been shown to be safe.
https://bnf.nice.org.uk/treatment-summaries/antidepressant-drugs/#other-antidepressant-drugs

45 C – Ramipril
Hyperkalaemia and other side-effects of ACE inhibitors (such as ramipril) are more common in those with impaired renal function.
https://bnf.nice.org.uk/drugs/ramipril/#monitoring-requirements

46 B – Ciclosporin
Purple grape juice is predicted to decrease exposure.
https://bnf.nice.org.uk/interactions/ciclosporin/

47 C – Bezafibrate
Muscle complaints are listed as a side effect of bezafibrate (uncommon).
https://bnf.nice.org.uk/drugs/bezafibrate/#side-effects

48 B – Isosorbide mononitrate
Flushing and headache are common or very common side effects for all nitrates.
https://bnf.nice.org.uk/drugs/isosorbide-mononitrate/

49 D – Pindolol
Pindolol, along with celiprolol hydrochloride, acebutolol, and oxprenolol

hydrochloride have intrinsic sympathomimetic activity; they tend to cause less bradycardia than the other beta-blockers and may also cause less coldness of the extremities.
https://bnf.nice.org.uk/treatment-summaries/beta-adrenoceptor-blocking-drugs/

50 **A – Citalopram**
QT interval prolongation is a common or very common side effect of citalopram.
https://bnf.nice.org.uk/drugs/citalopram/

51 **E – Stop lithium and to seek urgent medical attention**
Lithium salts have a narrow therapeutic/toxic ratio. Signs of intoxication require withdrawal of treatment and include increasing gastro-intestinal disturbances (vomiting, diarrhoea). With severe overdosage seizures, cardiac arrhythmias, blood pressure changes, circulatory failure, renal failure, coma and sudden death have been reported.
https://bnf.nice.org.uk/drugs/lithium-carbonate/#cautions

52 **A – Diclofenac**
Diclofenac increases the concentration of lithium.
https://bnf.nice.org.uk/interactions/lithium/

53 **E – Sertraline**
Sertraline, can safely be reduced and or stopped based on patient choice.
https://www.sps.nhs.uk/articles/choosing-an-antidepressant-for-people-with-coronary-heart-disease/#:~:text=SSRIs%20are%20the%20preferred%20antidepressants%20in%20CHD.%20Sertraline%2C,Mirtazapine%20is%20also%20a%20preferred%20antidepressant%20in%20CHD

54 **A – Buprenorphine**
Buprenorphine can be used as an adjunct in the treatment of opioid dependence.
https://bnf.nice.org.uk/drugs/buprenorphine/

55 **B – Ciprofloxacin**
Avoid quinolones in tendonitis / nerve damage.
https://bnf.nice.org.uk/drugs/ciprofloxacin/

56 **B – Migraine**
Migraine is the most likely working diagnosis as she reports unilateral symptoms and nausea is a common associated symptom.
https://cks.nice.org.uk/topics/migraine/

57 **B – Carbamazepine**
Should be brand prescribed as different formulations of oral preparations may vary in bioavailability.
https://bnf.nice.org.uk/drugs/carbamazepine/

58 **C – Prescribe fidaxomicin**
Fidaxomicin is indicated for the treatment of *C. difficile* infection.
https://bnf.nice.org.uk/drugs/fidaxomicin/

59 **A – Apply appropriate sunscreen if there is sun exposure**
Benzoyl peroxide should be applied 1 or 2 times a day after washing. If severe skin irritation occurs, the frequency of application should be reduced, or treatment temporarily discontinued or stopped. If sun exposure is unavoidable then an appropriate sunscreen or protective clothing should be used.
https://bnf.nice.org.uk/drugs/benzoyl-peroxide/#patient-and-carer-advice

60 **E – Refer the patient to the GP**
The patient is showing signs of pyelonephritis.
https://cks.nice.org.uk/topics/pyelonephritis-acute/diagnosis/diagnosis/

61 **C – Neuropathy**
Pyridoxine is indicated for the prophylaxis and treatment of isoniazid-induced neuropathy.
https://bnf.nice.org.uk/drugs/pyridoxine-hydrochloride/

62 **C – CRP**
CRP or C-reactive protein test is used to help diagnose conditions that cause inflammation. CRP is produced by the liver and a higher concentration of CRP is a sign of inflammation in the body.
https://www.nhsinform.scot/tests-and-treatments/blood-tests/common-blood-tests/

63 **E – Ritonavir**
Ritonavir is indicated for the treatment of HIV infection in combination with other antiretroviral drugs.
https://bnf.nice.org.uk/drugs/ritonavir/#indications-and-dose

64 **C – Metformin**
Metformin is contra-indicated in severe renal impairment and is cautioned for the risk of lactic acidosis.
https://bnf.nice.org.uk/drugs/metformin-hydrochloride/

65 **C – Metformin**
The patient is displaying signs of vitamin B12 deficiency. A common or very common side effect of metformin.
https://bnf.nice.org.uk/drugs/metformin-hydrochloride/#side-effects AND
https://bnf.nice.org.uk/treatment-summaries/anaemia-megaloblastic/

66 **D – Vitamin B12**
As above, the patient has signs of B12 deficiency. This can be treated by a course of vitamin B12.
https://bnf.nice.org.uk/drugs/metformin-hydrochloride/#side-effects AND
https://bnf.nice.org.uk/treatment-summaries/anaemia-megaloblastic/

67 **D – Stop the metformin and seek urgent advice from the GP**
The patient is showing signs of lactic acidosis and requires urgent medical attention. The metformin should be stopped.
https://bnf.nice.org.uk/drugs/metformin-hydrochloride/#side-effects AND
https://cks.nice.org.uk/topics/diabetes-type-2/prescribing-information/metformin/#adverse-effects

68 **B – Gliclazide**
Sulphonylureas, such as glicazide, can cause weight gain.
https://bnf.nice.org.uk/drugs/gliclazide/#cautions

69 **E – Pioglitazone**
Pioglitazone can exacerbate heart failure.
https://bnf.nice.org.uk/drugs/pioglitazone/#important-safety-information

70 **B – Empagliflozin**
Urinary disorders are listed as a common or very common side effect of empagliflozin.
https://bnf.nice.org.uk/drugs/empagliflozin/#side-effects

71 **D – Pioglitazone**
The symptoms the patient is experiencing suggest liver toxicity. Pioglitazone is listed as causing toxicity.
https://bnf.nice.org.uk/drugs/pioglitazone/

72 **E – Risedronate**
Atypical femoral fractures have been reported by patients receiving bisphosphonate treatment, mainly those receiving long-term treatment for osteoporosis. Discontinuation of bisphosphonate treatment such patients should be considered after an assessment of the benefits and risks of continued treatment.
https://bnf.nice.org.uk/drugs/risedronate-sodium/

73 **E – You may experience hypotension when initially prescribed this, your blood pressure should be monitored**
Low BP can occur at initiation of treatment, in addition you should counsel them on safe driving.
https://bnf.nice.org.uk/drugs/bromocriptine/#patient-and-carer-advice

74 **D – Methotrexate**
The BNF monograph for methotrexate cautions that bone marrow suppression can occur abruptly. The factors likely to increase toxicity include advanced age, renal impairment, and concomitant use with another anti-folate drug (e.g. trimethoprim). The manufacturer advises a clinically significant drop in white cell count or platelet count calls for immediate withdrawal of methotrexate and introduction of supportive therapy.
https://bnf.nice.org.uk/drugs/methotrexate/#cautions

75 **D – Methylprednisolone**
The patient is displaying symptoms for Cushing's Syndrome (https://www.nhs.uk/conditions/cushings-syndrome/). This is listed as a common or very common side effect of all corticosteroids.
https://bnf.nice.org.uk/drugs/methylprednisolone/#side-effects

High weighted answers | 127

76 **A – Being sensitive to cold and gaining weight**
Fatigue/lethargy, cold intolerance; weight gain and constipation are listed as symptoms of hypothyroidism.
https://cks.nice.org.uk/topics/hypothyroidism/diagnosis/diagnosis/

77 **D – <140/94**
A blood pressure reading of 140/90 or higher is an indication of hypertension.
https://cks.nice.org.uk/topics/hypertension/diagnosis/diagnosis/

78 **D – Ramipril 1.25mg tablet**
Dose for hypertension - Initially 1.25-2.5mg OD, increased if necessary up to 10mg once daily. Dose to be increased at intervals of 2-4 weeks.
https://bnf.nice.org.uk/drugs/ramipril/

79 **D – Blood Pressure, U&E and side effects**
Renal function and electrolytes should be checked after increasing the dose and monitored during treatment, (more frequently if side effects are present). Therefore check how patient is getting on with new medication and check blood pressure to titrate medication for optimal blood pressure results.
https://bnf.nice.org.uk/drugs/ramipril/

80 **C – The GP should request that the neurologist considers the most appropriate treatment for this patient given the fact she is of childbearing age. If the neurologist feels sodium valproate is the most appropriate treatment then they should sign the patient up to the Pregnancy Prevention Programme, explaining the risks associated with the medication.**
The GP should request that the neurologist considers the most appropriate treatment for this patient given the fact she is of childbearing age, since sodium valproate is unlicensed, it is not the most appropriate option. If the neurologist feels sodium valproate is the most appropriate treatment then they should sign the patient up to the Pregnancy Prevention Program, explaining the risks associated with the medication. To be noted that if the patient does become pregnant then sodium valproate is contraindicated.
https://www.gov.uk/drug-safety-update/valproate-pregnancy-prevention-programme-actions-required-now-from-gps-specialists-and-dispensers#:~:text=Valproate%20Pregnancy%20Prevention%20Programme:%20actions%20required AND https://bnf.nice.org.uk/drugs/sodium-valproate/#prescribing-and-dispensing-information

81 **C** – Citalopram and escitalopram have a potential to cause QT interval prolongation. Elderly patients have a higher exposure due to age related decline in metabolism and elimination. The maximum dose of both medicines has therefore been restricted in patients older than 65 years.

Citalopram
Adults max dose: Citalopram 40mg OD.
Adults over 65 years: Citalopram 20mg OD

Escitalopram
Adults max dose: Escitalopram 20mg OD
Adults over 65 years: Escitalopram 10mg OD

Therefore dose should be reduced to Citalopram 20mg OD not Escitalopram 20mg OD.

https://www.gov.uk/drug-safety-update/citalopram-and-escitalopram-qt-interval-prolongation#:~:text=Citalopram.%20The%20data%20for%20citalopram%20include%20double-blind

82 **C** – Book in with GP for review - it has been a year since patient last had this medication issued and will need to be reviewed by GP to see if medication is appropriate
Last had a year ago therefore requires further review from GP. It is correct to note that zopiclone can be given once daily at bedtime for up to 4 weeks only. Prolonged use can result in withdrawal symptoms.
https://bnf.nice.org.uk/drugs/zopiclone/

83 **A** – Carbamazepine should be withdrawn immediately in cases of aggravated liver dysfunction or acute liver disease. Patients, or their carers, should be told how to recognise the signs of blood, liver or skin disorders, and advised to seek immediate medical attention if symptoms such as fever, as, mouth ulcers, bruising or bleeding develop.
https://bnf.nice.org.uk/drugs/carbamazepine/#cautions

84 **C – Propranolol**
Lipophilic beta-blockers such as propranolol and metaprolol are

associated with reduced excretion of melatonin resulting in nightmares.
https://bnf.nice.org.uk/treatment-summaries/beta-adrenoceptor-blocking-drugs/
https://www.ncbi.nlm.nih.gov/pmc/articles/PMC7914867/

85 **B – Dry mouth, constipation and urinary retention**
Anticholinergics block acetylcholine which reduces the amount of fluids being made resulting in dry mouth, constipation and urinary retention.
https://bnf.nice.org.uk/drugs/amitriptyline-hydrochloride/#side-effects

86 **B – 10mg TDS**
As per BNF - Nausea and vomiting in palliative care - 10mg three times a day.
https://bnf.nice.org.uk/drugs/metoclopramide-hydrochloride/#indications-and-dose

87 **D – Serum lipids and weight**
As per BNF - Blood lipids and weight should be measured at baseline.
https://bnf.nice.org.uk/drugs/olanzapine/#monitoring-requirements

88 **D – The correct dose of diclofenac for muscular back pain is 75mg/mr tablet - Take ONE three times a day**
As per BNF - Pain and inflammation of musculoskeletal disorders: By using modified-release medicines: Adult: 75mg - 1-2 times a day, alternatively 100mg once daily.
https://bnf.nice.org.uk/drugs/diclofenac/

89 **D – The quantity of pregabalin is incorrect**
Pregabalin is a schedule 3 controlled drug, the maximum quantity should not exceed 30 days. Therefore, the maximum quantity should be 60.
MEP - Controlled Drugs - Prescription requirements for Schedule 2 and 3 Controlled Drugs

90 **D – 30%**
According to the BNF, when switching from modified-release levodopa to dispersible co-beneldopa the dose should be reduced by 30%.
https://bnf.nice.org.uk/drugs/co-beneldopa/#prescribing-and-dispensing-information

91 B – Gliclazide
As per BNF - The risk of hypoglycaemia associated with sulphonylureas should be discussed with the patient, especially when concomitant glucose-lowering drugs are prescribed.
https://bnf.nice.org.uk/drugs/gliclazide/

92 F – Metformin
Metformin is used in the treatment of type II diabetes, however it is also used for the treatment of PCOS.
https://bnf.nice.org.uk/drugs/metformin-hydrochloride/#indications-and-dose

93 E – Linagliptin
Linagliptin is used in the treatment of type II diabetes. Its method of action is to inhibit dipeptidylpeptidase-4 to increase insulin secretion and lower glucagon secretion.
https://bnf.nice.org.uk/drugs/linagliptin/#drug-action

94 A – Empagliflozin (risk of diabetic ketoacidosis, see MHRA advice)
https://bnf.nice.org.uk/drugs/empagliflozin/#important-safety-information

95 F – Metformin
You should avoid using metformin if eGFR<30 due to risk of lactic acidosis.
https://bnf.nice.org.uk/drugs/metformin-hydrochloride/#indications-and-dose

96 D – Advise patient to see her GP immediately for review and blood test
Due to risk of neutropenia and agranulocytosis with carbimazole. Sore throat and symptoms suggest an infection and needs to be seen by the GP immediately. Blood tests need to be undertaken to see if any clinical evidence of infection.
https://bnf.nice.org.uk/drugs/carbimazole/#important-safety-information

97 C – Measure TSH levels every 3 months until a stable level has been achieved then yearly thereafter
Consider measuring TSH levels every 3 months until a stable level has been achieved, then yearly thereafter. Monitoring free thyroxine should be considered in those who continue to be symptomatic.
https://bnf.nice.org.uk/drugs/levothyroxine-sodium/#monitoring-requirements

98 **B – Alendronic acid tablets**
As per BNF - manufacturer advises tablets should be swallowed whole. Doses should be taken with plenty of water while sitting or standing, on an empty stomach at least 30 minutes before breakfast (or another oral medicine); patient should stand or sit upright for at least 30 minutes after administration.
https://bnf.nice.org.uk/drugs/alendronic-acid/#directions-for-administration

99 **A – Advise patient to continue with what she is currently doing as it is self-limiting and should resolve soon. If it doesn't within 5 days, she should return.**
Only treat if severe. Bacterial conjunctivitis is usually unilateral and also self-limiting. 65% resolve by day five. As per patients symptoms - doesn't seem severe.
https://cks.nice.org.uk/topics/conjunctivitis-infective/

100 **D – Impetigo**
Based on the description of reddish sore and orange, honey-coloured crusty patches - it is most likely impetigo.
https://cks.nice.org.uk/topics/impetigo/

101 **E – False positive urinary glucose tests have been reported**
Laboratory tests can be impacted
https://bnf.nice.org.uk/drugs/cefalexin/#effect-on-laboratory-tests

102 **B – Long term oral corticosteroid is usually recommended at the lowest dose possible. Patients should be monitored for osteoporosis.**
As per BNF - long-term oral corticosteroid is not usually recommended, however in some patients this may need to be continued when withdrawal following an exacerbation is not possible, in this context, the lowest dose possible should be used. Patients should be monitored for osteoporosis and given appropriate prophylaxis.
https://bnf.nice.org.uk/treatment-summaries/chronic-obstructive-pulmonary-disease/

103 **C – H-Pylori**
As per BNF - treatment for H-Pylori.
https://bnf.nice.org.uk/treatment-summaries/helicobacter-pylori-infection/

104 **C – Lansoprazole 30mg BD for 7 days**
Metronidazole 400mg BD for 7 days
Clarithromycin 500mg BD for 7 days
As per BNF - treatment for H-Pylori with patients who have a penicillin allergy.
https://bnf.nice.org.uk/treatment-summaries/helicobacter-pylori-infection/

105 **E – Simvastatin**
As per NICE guidelines - Clarithromycin should not be given at the same time as simvastatin - when taken together they may significantly increase the blood levels of simvastatin. This can lead to liver damage and a rare but serious condition called rhabdomyolosis which involves the breakdown of skeletal muscle tissue.
https://cks.nice.org.uk/topics/bronchiectasis/prescribing-information/clarithromycin/

106 **H – Norethisterone**
As per BNF - Postponement of menstruation - females of child-bearing potential - 5mg three times a day to be started three days before expected onset.
https://bnf.nice.org.uk/drugs/norethisterone/

107 **A – Desogestrel**
As per BNF - Desogestrel is a progesterone only pill that is to be taken daily - 75mcg daily, dose to be taken at the same time each day, starting on day 1 of cycle then continuously, if administration delayed for 12 hours or more it should be regarded as a 'missed pill.'
https://bnf.nice.org.uk/drugs/desogestrel/

108 **G – Levonorgestrel**
As per BNF - Levonorgestrel for emergency contraception - 1.5mg for 1 dose, taken as soon as possible after coitus, preferably within 12 hours and no later than after 72 hours (may also be used between 72 - 96 hours after coitus but efficacy decreases with time).
https://bnf.nice.org.uk/drugs/levonorgestrel/#indications-and-dose

109 **F – Intra-uterine contraceptive device**
As per MHRA advice (June 2015) uterine perforation most often occurs during insertion of IUD but might not be detected until sometime later. The risk of uterine perforation is increased when the device is inserted up to 36 weeks postpartum or in patients who are breastfeeding.
https://www.gov.uk/drug-safety-update/intrauterine-contraception-uterine-perforation-updated-information-on-risk-factors

High weighted answers | 133

110 **D – Ethinylestradiol 30mcg/Levonorgestrel 50mcg**
As per BNF - there is an increased risk of venous thromboembolic disease in users of combined hormonal contraceptives particularly during first year and possibly after restarting combined hormonal contraceptives following a break of four weeks or more. In all cases the risk of venous thromboembolism increases with age and in the presence of other risk factors such as obesity. The risk also depends on the type of progesterone and oestrogen dose.
https://bnf.nice.org.uk/drugs/ethinylestradiol-with-levonorgestrel/#cautions

111 **A – Androgenetic alopecia in men**
As per BNF - for androgenetic alopecia in men - given at a dose of 1mg once daily, continuous use for 3 - 6 months is required before benefit is seen and effects are reversed 6 - 12 months after treatment is discontinued.
https://bnf.nice.org.uk/drugs/finasteride/

112 **E –Replens® MD moisturiser**
As per BNF - for vaginal atrophy, patient can use topical oestrogen such as estradiol pessaries, vaginal rings or estriol pessaries, cream and gel. Non-hormonal preparations can also be used such as vaginal moisturisers. In the list given the most appropriate from the list is Replens® MD moisturiser which is a vaginal moisturiser to help with the vaginal dryness the patient is complaining of. There was no option for the topical oestrogen in the list however that too could be used for treatment of vaginal atrophy.
https://bnf.nice.org.uk/treatment-summaries/vaginal-and-vulval-conditions/

113 **E –Tadalafil 5mg**
As per BNF - Tadalafil is a longer acting drug. It can be used as required, but can also be used as a regular daily dose to allow for spontaneous (rather than scheduled) sexual activity or in those who have frequent sexual activity.
https://bnf.nice.org.uk/drugs/tadalafil/#indications-and-dose

114 **C – Metronidazole vaginal gel 0.5% nightly for 5 nights**
As per BNF and guidelines -Advised during pregnancy to avoid high dose regimens of metronidazole.
Metronidazole 400mg QDS is the incorrect dose, usually 400mg

BD for 7 days. Metronidazole 4g STAT is too high. Clotrimazole and fluconazole to be used in fungal infections not bacterial.
https://bnf.nice.org.uk/drugs/metronidazole/#pregnancy

115 **B – If a pregnant woman develops vulvovaginal candidasis she will need a shorter duration of treatment to ensure safety of the foetus**
As per BNF - Pregnant women need a longer duration of treatment usually about 7 days to clear the infection.
https://bnf.nice.org.uk/treatment-summaries/vaginal-and-vulval-conditions/

116 **E – Simvastatin**
Statin medications to be offered to reduce the risk of CVD
https://cks.nice.org.uk/topics/lipid-modification-cvd-prevention/prescribing-information/statins/ AND *https://cks.nice.org.uk/topics/cvd-risk-assessment-management/management/cvd-risk-assessment/#:~:text=This%20means%20that%20you%20have%20a%2020%20in%20100%20chance*

117 **D – Peripheral oedema**
Peripheral oedema is listed as a common or very common side effect of amlodipine.
https://bnf.nice.org.uk/drugs/amlodipine/#side-effects

118 **C – They can cause a persistent dry cough as a side effect**
Cough is listed as a common or very common side effect of ramipril.
https://bnf.nice.org.uk/drugs/ramipril/#side-effects

119 **A – Aspirin**
As per NICE guidance - Aspirin alone or in combination with other drugs is the first step in the medical management of STEMI.
visual-summary-stemi-pdf-8900623405 (nice.org.uk)

120 **A – Bisoprolol**
As per BNF - For long-term prevention of chest pain in patients with stable angina, a beta-blocker such as bisoprolol should be given as first-line therapy.
https://bnf.nice.org.uk/treatment-summaries/stable-angina/#aims-of-treatment

121 E – Salmeterol
Salmeterol is a long-acting beta2 agonist, while salbutamol is a short-acting beta2 agonist.
https://bnf.nice.org.uk/treatment-summaries/asthma-chronic/

122 D – Oral candidiasis
Oral candidiasis is a common or very common side effect of beclometasone.
https://bnf.nice.org.uk/drugs/beclometasone-dipropionate/#side-effects

123 C – Salbutamol
A short-acting beta2 agonist such as salbutamol should be used for symptom relief of asthma.
https://bnf.nice.org.uk/treatment-summaries/asthma-chronic/

124 E – Muscarinic receptor antagonist
Ipratropium is a muscarinic receptor antagonist.
https://cks.nice.org.uk/topics/chronic-obstructive-pulmonary-disease/prescribing-information/muscarinic-antagonists/

125 A – Clenil® inhaler
Next stepwise treatment is to initiate a steroid based inhaler
https://cks.nice.org.uk/topics/asthma/management/newly-diagnosed-asthma/ AND *https://www.brit-thoracic.org.uk/quality-improvement/clinical-resources/asthma/*

126 B – Metformin
Metformin is first-line treatment for adult patients with type II diabetes.
https://cks.nice.org.uk/topics/diabetes-type-2/management/management-adults/

127 D – Levothyroxine
As per BNF – Levothyroxine is first-line treatment for hypothyroidism.
https://bnf.nice.org.uk/treatment-summaries/hypothyroidism/

128 A – Arrythmias
Arrythmias are listed as a side effect of levothyroxine – frequency not known.
https://bnf.nice.org.uk/drugs/levothyroxine-sodium/#side-effects

129 D – Osteoporosis
Usually the risk is of osteoporosis with over treatment of thyroid medication or hyperthyroidism, the question states over-replacement (not side effect)
https://www.btf-thyroid.org/thyroid-disorders-and-osteoporosis#ost5

130 E – Always carry a steroid treatment card
The other options are incorrect.
https://bnf.nice.org.uk/drugs/hydrocortisone/#patient-and-carer-advice

131 A – Agranulocytosis
As per BNF – Agranulocytosis is listed as a side effect of carbimazole – frequency not known. Important safety information - Manufacturer advises of the importance of recognising bone marrow suppression induced by carbimazole and the need to stop treatment promptly.
https://bnf.nice.org.uk/drugs/carbimazole/#side-effects

132 E – Ramipril
As per NICE guidance – Commence with ACE due to patient's history of diabetes
https://www.nice.org.uk/guidance/ng136/chapter/Recommendations#treating-and-monitoring-hypertension

133 C – INR levels
For warfarin it is essential that the INR should be determined either daily or on alternate days in early stages of treatment, then at longer intervals (depending on the patient's response, graduating up to every 12 weeks.
https://bnf.nice.org.uk/drugs/warfarin-sodium/#monitoring-requirements

134 C – Aspirin, clopidogrel, ramipril, bisoprolol, atorvastatin
As per BNF - aspirin, clopidogrel, ramipril, bisoprolol, atorvastatin
https://bnf.nice.org.uk/treatment-summaries/acute-coronary-syndromes/

135 E – Spironolactone
As per BNF, it can raise potassium levels
Spironolactone | Drugs | BNF | NICE
https://bnf.nice.org.uk/drugs/spironolactone/#side-effects

136 E – Nitrofurantoin

As per NICE CKS - Prescribe an immediate antibiotic, taking into account recent urine culture and susceptibility testing results, any recent antibiotic use, local antimicrobial resistance patterns, and any contraindications. Options include, Nitrofurantoin 100 mg modified-release twice a day for 7 days.
https://cks.nice.org.uk/topics/urinary-tract-infection-lower-women/ management/asymptomatic-bacteriuria-in-pregnancy/

137 C – CRB-65

Use CRB-65 and clinical judgement to aid diagnosis
https://cks.nice.org.uk/topics/chest-infections-adult/management/ community-acquired-pneumonia/

138 A – Advise self-care and offer amoxicillin

Advise the person on self-care strategies such as rest, adequate fluid intake, and the use of simple analgesia for symptomatic relief. For a patient with a CRB-65 score of 1 or 2, oral amoxicillin 500 mg three times a day for 5 days can be prescribed.
https://cks.nice.org.uk/topics/chest-infections-adult/management/ community-acquired-pneumonia/

139 C – Diarrhoea

As per BNF - Diarrhoea is a common or very common side effect of all penicillins.
https://bnf.nice.org.uk/drugs/amoxicillin/#side-effects

140 D – Miconazole

If the infection is mild and localized, a topical antifungal treatment for 14 days can be prescribed. Miconazole oral gel is recommended as first-line treatment.
https://cks.nice.org.uk/topics/candida-oral/management/adults-young-people-not-immunocompromised/

141 A – Fluconazole

If the infection is extensive or severe either fluconazole 50mg a day for at least 14 days can be prescribed or the patient should be referred for specialist advice.
https://cks.nice.org.uk/topics/candida-oral/management/adults-young-people-not-immunocompromised/

142 C – Bacterial vaginosis

As per NICE CKS – the other options can be eliminated by differential diagnosis.
https://cks.nice.org.uk/topics/bacterial-vaginosis/diagnosis/differential-diagnosis/

143 C – Metronidazole

As per NICE CKS - oral metronidazole 400 mg twice a day for 5 to 7 days can be prescribed for women who are not pregnant.
https://cks.nice.org.uk/topics/bacterial-vaginosis/management/women-who-are-not-pregnant/

144 E – Vancomycin

NICE recommends vancomycin 125 mg orally four times a day for 10 days for an initial episode of non-severe *clostridioides difficile*.
https://cks.nice.org.uk/topics/diarrhoea-antibiotic-associated/management/diarrhoea-antibiotic-associated/#suspected-or-confirmed-clostridiodes-difficile-infections AND https://bnf.nice.org.uk/drugs/vancomycin/#indications-and-dose

145 D – Sertraline

Drug treatment would only be commenced after non-medication treatment options had been tried. NICE recommend a SSRI as first-line treatment.
https://cks.nice.org.uk/topics/generalized-anxiety-disorder/management/management/

146 C – Hyperglycaemia

Hyperglycaemia is a common or very common side effect of all antipsychotic drugs.
https://bnf.nice.org.uk/drugs/olanzapine/#side-effects

147 E – Venlafaxine

Venlafaxine a serotonin and noradrenaline re-uptake inhibitor (SNRI) and is indicated for major depression.
https://bnf.nice.org.uk/drugs/venlafaxine/#indications-and-dose

148 A – Dry mouth

As per BNF – Dry mouth is a side effect of amitriptyline – frequency not known.
https://bnf.nice.org.uk/drugs/amitriptyline-hydrochloride/#side-effects

149 **B – Take 10mg OD for up to 4 weeks**
Zolpidem is indicated for the short-term treatment of insomnia. Maximum period of treatment is 4 weeks.
https://bnf.nice.org.uk/drugs/zolpidem-tartrate/#indications-and-dose

150 **D – Take one tablet at the onset of a migraine, if there is no symptom relief then another tablet can be taken after 2 hours**
Sumatriptan is not indicated for epilepsy, it can be taken by adults between the ages of 18 and 65 years. It is not used as a preventative treatment. Maximum daily dose is 2 tablets.
https://www.medicines.org.uk/emc/product/8337/pil AND
https://bnf.nice.org.uk/drugs/sumatriptan/#indications-and-dose

151 **D – Treatment of bipolar disorder**
As per BNF – Lithium is indicated for the treatment and prophylaxis of mania, bipolar disorder, recurrent depression and aggressive or self-harming behaviour.
https://bnf.nice.org.uk/drugs/lithium-carbonate/#indications-and-dose

152 **A – Lithium drug levels, eGFR, thyroid levels**
Lithium has a narrow therapeutic/toxic ratio and should not be prescribed unless monitoring serum-lithium concentrations can be monitored. Manufacturer also advises monitoring of eGFR, and thyroid function every 6 months during treatment as a minimum.
https://bnf.nice.org.uk/drugs/lithium-carbonate/#monitoring-requirements

153 **C – Memory impairment**
Long term use of lithium associated with memory impairment.
https://bnf.nice.org.uk/drugs/lithium-carbonate/#side-effects

154 **B – 0.4 – 1mmol/L**
A routine serum-lithium concentration of 0.4–1 mmol/litre (lower end of the range for maintenance therapy and elderly patients) is recommended. A concentration of 0.8–1 mmol/litre is recommended for acute episodes of mania, and for patients who have previously relapsed or have sub-syndromal symptoms.
https://bnf.nice.org.uk/drugs/lithium-carbonate/#monitoring-requirements

155 **D – Maintain adequate fluid intake, avoid dietary changes which reduce or increase sodium intake**
Patients taking lithium should be advised to avoid changes to their sodium intake and ensure adequate fluid intake.
https://bnf.nice.org.uk/drugs/lithium-carbonate/#patient-and-carer-advice

156 **D – Mirtazapine (side effect is sedative properties), could consider trazodone however, mirtazapine should be considered first.**
https://bnf.nice.org.uk/drugs/mirtazapine/

157 **B – Fluoxetine**
Fluoxetine has a long half-life that needs to be considered when adjusting dosage. It is the preferred antidepressant for treating moderate and severe depression in children and young people as it is the only antidepressant where the benefits outweigh the risks.
https://bnf.nice.org.uk/drugs/fluoxetine/#indications-and-dose AND https://cks.nice.org.uk/topics/depression-in-children/prescribing-information/fluoxetine/

158 **E – Paroxetine**
An SSRI type of medication with a short half-life and associated with a higher risk of withdrawal symptoms
https://cks.nice.org.uk/topics/depression/management/ongoing-management/#switching-antidepressants
https://www.medicines.org.uk/emc/product/537/smpc#gref

159 **F – Sertraline**
Sertraline is known to be the first choice antidepressant in those with a history of cardiac disease.
https://bnf.nice.org.uk/drugs/sertraline/
https://www.sps.nhs.uk/articles/choosing-an-antidepressant-for-people-with-coronary-heart-disease/
https://www.nice.org.uk/guidance/ng222

160 **D – Mirtazapine**
Mirtazapine is a presynaptic alpha2-adrenoreceptor antagonist which increases central noradrenergic and serotonergic neurotransmission.
https://bnf.nice.org.uk/drugs/mirtazapine/#drug-action

161 E – Flucloxacillin
As per NICE CKS – Flucloxacillin is first line treatment for the management of cellulitis in primary care.
https://cks.nice.org.uk/topics/cellulitis-acute/management/management/#oral-antibiotics-in-primary-care

162 E – Flucloxacillin
Cholestatic jaundice and hepatitis can occur up to two months after treatment with flucloxacillin. Risk factors are increasing age and treatment for more than 2 weeks.
https://bnf.nice.org.uk/drugs/flucloxacillin/#important-safety-information

163 F – Gentamicin
MHRA advises that the use of aminoglycosides is associated with rare cases of ototoxicity. BNF also lists nephrotoxicity as an important side effect to consider.
https://bnf.nice.org.uk/drugs/gentamicin/#important-safety-information

164 C – Ciprofloxacin
The CSM has warned that there is a risk that quinolones may induce convulsions in patients.
https://bnf.nice.org.uk/drugs/ciprofloxacin/#important-safety-information

165 C – Ciprofloxacin
Tendon damage has been reported in some patients receiving quinolones. The rupture may occur with 48 hours of treatment starting.
https://bnf.nice.org.uk/drugs/ciprofloxacin/#important-safety-information

166 C – Clopidogrel
As per NICE CKS – Clopidogrel is the standard treatment, 75 mg daily.
https://cks.nice.org.uk/topics/stroke-tia/management/secondary-prevention-following-stroke-tia/

167 D – Digoxin
Digoxin is indicated for atrial fibrillation and atrial flutter. For plasma-digoxin concentration, blood should be taken at least 6 hours after a dose.
https://bnf.nice.org.uk/drugs/digoxin/#indications-and-dose

168 A – Amiodarone
As per BNF – Monitoring requirements for amiodarone are: a chest x-ray is required prior to treatment; liver function tests both prior to treatment and every 6 months; thyroid function both prior to treatment and every 6 months.
https://bnf.nice.org.uk/drugs/amiodarone-hydrochloride/#monitoring-requirements

169 F – Furosemide
Furosemide is indicated for oedema.
https://bnf.nice.org.uk/drugs/furosemide/#indications-and-dose

170 A – Amiodarone
These side-effects can occur at any time during treatment with amiodarone and also in the months after stopping treatment.
https://bnf.nice.org.uk/drugs/amiodarone-hydrochloride/#side-effects

171 E – Metformin
As per NICE CKS – Metformin is used to treat type II diabetes at an initial dose of 500mg daily.
https://cks.nice.org.uk/topics/diabetes-type-2/prescribing-information/metformin/

172 B – Dulaglutide
As per NICE CKS – Dulaglutide is 1 of 6 GLP-1 receptor agonists available and is self-administered by subcutaneous injection once a week.
https://cks.nice.org.uk/topics/diabetes-type-2/prescribing-information/glp-1-receptor-agonists/

173 G – Pioglitazone
MHRA advise pioglitazone should not be used in patients with heart failure or a history of heart failure.
https://bnf.nice.org.uk/drugs/pioglitazone/#important-safety-information

174 F – Ozempic
https://www.gov.uk/government/news/mhra-warns-of-unsafe-fake-weight-loss-pens

175 **A – Canagliflozin**

As per NICE CKS – Canagliflozin in 1 of 4 SGLT-2 inhibitors available. Prior to treatment, you need to check whether a patient is at increased risk of diabetic ketoacidosis, for example if they have had a previous episode or are following a low carbohydrate diet.

https://cks.nice.org.uk/topics/diabetes-type-2/prescribing-information/sglt-2-inhibitors/

Medium weighted answers

176 A – Finasteride
Finasteride metabolises testosterone into the more potent androgen, dihydrotestosterone. Women of childbearing age should avoid handling crushed or broken tablets.
https://bnf.nice.org.uk/drugs/finasteride/#handling-and-storage

177 B – Onset of nausea
Onset of nausea is not listed as a reason for stopping oral contraception immediately in the SmPC. Nausea is a very common side effect of Microgynon 30
https://www.medicines.org.uk/emc/product/1130/smpc

178 B – Do not crush or chew
Modified released preparations should not be crushed or chewed as this will damage the modified release coating.
https://www.medicines.org.uk/emc/product/9245/smpc#gref

179 D – 120 hours
As per BNF treatment summary - A copper intra-uterine contraceptive device can be inserted up to 5 days (120 hours) after the first UPSI in a natural menstrual cycle.
https://bnf.nice.org.uk/treatment-summaries/emergency-contraception/

180 B – Two to three times a day
The cream should be applied thinly two or three a day and rubbed in gently. Treatment should continue until the symptoms disappear.
https://www.medicines.org.uk/emc/product/2206/smpc#gref

181 **H –Senna**
Senna is a stimulant laxative which can increase intestinal motility and often causes abdominal cramps. It should be avoided in cases of intestinal obstruction. Co-danthramer and co-danthrusate have similar properties but are restricted to the use of the terminally ill.
https://bnf.nice.org.uk/treatment-summaries/constipation/

182 **B – Docusate sodium**
Docusate sodium is a faecal softner which acts by decreasing surface tension and increasing penetration of the faecal mass by intestinal fluid.
https://bnf.nice.org.uk/treatment-summaries/constipation/

183 **G – Macrogol**
Macrogols are inert polymers of ethylene glycol which sequester fluid in the bowel.
https://bnf.nice.org.uk/treatment-summaries/constipation/

184 **E – Linaclotide**
Linaclotide is a guanylate cyclase-C receptor agonist. It is licensed for the treatment of moderate to severe irritable bowel syndrome.
https://bnf.nice.org.uk/treatment-summaries/constipation/

185 **C – Ispaghula husk**
In patients with opioid-induced constipation bulk-forming laxatives such as ispaghula husk should be avoided.
https://bnf.nice.org.uk/treatment-summaries/constipation/

186 **D – Lactulose**
Lactulose is useful in the treatment of hepatic encephalopathy as it produces an osmotic diarrhoea of low faecal pH and inhibits the development of ammonia-producing organisms.
https://bnf.nice.org.uk/treatment-summaries/constipation/

187 **A – Co-danthramer**
Co-danthramer and co-danthrusate are restricted to the treatment of constipation in terminally ill patients due to potential carcinogenicity.
https://bnf.nice.org.uk/treatment-summaries/constipation/

188 D – Lactulose
A bulk-forming laxative is the first choice for a pregnant patient but an osmotic laxative, like lactulose, can also be used. Senna should be avoided near term or in cases of unstable pregnancy.
https://bnf.nice.org.uk/treatment-summaries/constipation/

189 C – Diffuse mucosal inflammation
In Crohn's disease, the inflammation extends through all layers, whereas in ulcerative colitis, the inflammation is diffuse and doesn't affect all layers.
https://bnf.nice.org.uk/treatment-summaries/crohns-disease/

190 H – Salbutamol
As per SPC - The active ingredient in Ventolin Evohaler® is salbutamol.
https://www.medicines.org.uk/emc/product/850/smpc#gref

191 F – Glycopyrronium bromide
As per SPC - The active ingredient in Seebri Breezhaler® is glycopyrronium bromide.
https://www.medicines.org.uk/emc/product/2840/smpc#gref

192 A – Beclomethasone dipropionate with formoterol fumarate and glycopyrronium bromide
As per SPC - The active ingredients in Trimbow® are beclomethasone dipropionate with formoterol fumarate and glycopyrronium bromide.
https://www.medicines.org.uk/emc/product/761/smpc

193 C – Fluticasone with formoterol
As per SPC - The active ingredients in Flutiform® are fluticasone with formoterol.
Rationale: see SmPC - https://www.medicines.org.uk/emc/product/7649/smpc

194 E – Fluticasone with umeclidinium bromide and vilanterol
As per SPC - The active ingredients in Trelegy Ellipta® are fluticasone with umeclidinium bromide and vilanterol.
https://www.medicines.org.uk/emc/product/8666

Medium weighted answers | 147

195 D – Fluticasone with salmeterol
As per SPC - The active ingredients in Seretide Accuhaler® are fluticasone with salmeterol.
https://www.medicines.org.uk/emc/product/5504/smpc

196 D – Spacer devices remove the need for coordination
Spacer devices remove the need for coordination between actuation and inhalation by reducing the velocity of the aerosol.
https://bnf.nice.org.uk/treatment-summaries/respiratory-system-inhaled-drug-delivery/#spacer-devices

197 D – Montelukast
NICE recommend adding a leukotriene receptor antagonist whereas BTS suggests adding a long acting beta agonist.
https://www.nice.org.uk/guidance/ng80

198 A – Alimemazine
All old generation antihistamines cause sedation as they cross the blood brain barrieir but alimemazine and promethazine are more sedating than chlorphenamine and cyclizine. Ceterizine and loratadine are newer generation antihistamines that are known as 'non sedating' as they penetrate the blood brain barrier only to a slight extent.
https://bnf.nice.org.uk/treatment-summaries/antihistamines-allergen-immunotherapy-and-allergic-emergencies/

199 A – 300 micrograms
As per BNF treatment summary – See table.
https://bnf.nice.org.uk/treatment-summaries/antihistamines-allergen-immunotherapy-and-allergic-emergencies/#dose-of-intramuscular-injection-of-adrenaline-epinephrine-for-the-emergency-treatment-of-anaphylaxis-by-healthcare-professionals

200 D – All of the above
As per SPC – See instructions for use in patient information leaflet.
https://www.medicines.org.uk/emc/files/pil.6975.pdf

201 C – 5mg daily, before conception until week 12 of pregnancy

As per BNF – The dose for women wishing to become pregnant and at high risk of neural tube defects in their baby is 5mg daily, before conception until week 12 of pregnancy.
https://bnf.nice.org.uk/drugs/folic-acid/#indications-and-dose

202 C – Hypocalcaemia
Hypoparathyroidism, leading to hypocalcaemia can cause paraesthesia in fingertips, toes and lips.
https://www.nhs.uk/conditions/hypoparathyroidism/

203 D – Hypomagnaesemia
Hypercalcaemia, hypokalaemia and hypomagesaemia can all increase the risk of digoxin toxicity.
https://bnf.nice.org.uk/drugs/digoxin/

204 E – Sertaline 50mg OD, started 2 weeks ago
Key signs of hyponatraemia are weakness, vomiting and confusion. Hyponatraemia can be caused by antidepressants such as sertraline.
https://bnf.nice.org.uk/drugs/sertraline/#side-effects

205 A – Ferric carboxymaltose
As per BNF treatment summary - Iron can be administered parenterally as iron dextran, iron sucrose, ferric carboxymaltose, or ferric derisomaltose.
https://bnf.nice.org.uk/treatment-summaries/anaemia-iron-deficiency/

206 E – Metronidazole
An adverse effect of metronidazole is a furred tongue.
https://www.medicines.org.uk/emc/product/12817/smpc

207 A – Can affect performance of driving
All antimuscarinics an affect the performance of skilled tasks such as driving.
https://bnf.nice.org.uk/drugs/solifenacin-succinate/#patient-and-carer-advice AND https://bnf.nice.org.uk/treatment-summaries/constipation/

208 A – Alverine citrate and ispaghula husk
In IBS patients, lactulose should not be used as first line laxative as it

may cause bloating. Linaclotide is used in IBS patients who have not responded to laxatives from different classes and have had constipation for at least 12 months – which is not the case for our patient. Amitriptyline (unlicensed) is used in IBS as a second line option in IBS patients who have not responded to antispasmodics and laxatives. Loperamide is an anti-motility drug for the relief of diarrhoea.
https://bnf.nice.org.uk/treatment-summaries/constipation/

209 **D – Obesity Class II**
In Caucasian individuals, overweight and obesity is defined as below:
- Healthy weight: BMI 18.5 – 24.9kg/m2
- Overweight: BMI 25 – 29.9kg/m2
- Obesity Class I: BMI 30 – 34.9kg/m2
- Obesity Class II: BMI 35 – 39.9kg/m2
- Obesity Class III: BMI 40kg/m2 or more.

https://www.who.int/europe/news-room/fact-sheets/item/a-healthy-lifestyle---who-recommendations

210 **B – Risk of dizziness**
For Saxenda® patients and carers should be cautioned on the increased risk of dizziness, particularly in the first 3 months of treatment. This can affect driving and performance of skilled tasks.
https://www.medicines.org.uk/emc/product/2313

211 **A – Clopidogrel**
Oesophageal varices are dilated collateral blood vessels that develop as a complication of portal hypertension, usually in the setting of cirrhosis. In Europe, the major cause of cirrhosis is alcoholic liver disease. Rupture of oesophageal varices can cause life-threatening bleeding. Antiplatelets, such as clopidogrel, can make bleeding worse so should be withheld immediately.
https://bnf.nice.org.uk/drugs/clopidogrel/#side-effect

212 **D – Terlipressin IV**
Terlipressin should be offered to patients with suspected variceal bleeding at presentation. Stop treatment after definitive haemostasis has been achieved.
https://bnf.nice.org.uk/drugs/terlipressin-acetate/

213 B – Propranolol

The patient has already experienced variceal bleeding so would require secondary prophylaxis. For primary prophylaxis, non-cardioselective beta-blockers (propranolol first line, carveilol or nadolol are alternative) is the recommended treatment. For secondary prophylaxis, non-cardioselective beta-blockers (propranolol or nadolol) and variceal band ligation combination therapy are recommended.
https://www.nice.org.uk/guidance/CG141/chapter/Recommendations#management-of-variceal-bleeding,
https://bnf.nice.org.uk/drugs/propranolol-hydrochloride/#indications-and-dose,
https://bnf.nice.org.uk/drugs/carvedilol/#indications-and-dose

214 D – Thiopurine methyltransferase (TPMT) activity

Thiopurine methyltransferase (TPMT) metabolises thiopurine drugs (azathioprine, mercaptopurine, tioguanine); the risk of myelosuppression is increased in patients with reduced activity of the enzyme, particularly for the few individuals in whom TPMT activity is undetectable. Manufacturer advises consider measuring TPMT activity before starting azathioprine, mercaptopurine, or tioguanine therapy.
https://bnf.nice.org.uk/drugs/azathioprine/#pre-treatment-screening

215 C – Methotrexate

In Crohn's disease, add on treatment is prescribed if there are two or more inflammatory exacerbations in a 12-month period, or the corticosteroid dose cannot be reduced. Azathioprine or mercaptopurine (unlicensed with mercaptopurine) can be added to a corticosteroid or budesonide to induce remission. In patients who cannot tolerate azathioprine or mercaptopurine or in whom thiopurine methyltransferase (TPMT) activity is deficient, methotrexate can be added to a corticosteroid.
https://bnfc.nice.org.uk/treatment-summaries/crohns-disease/

216 B – Infliximab

Under specialist supervision, the tumour necrosis factor-alpha inhibitors adalimumab and infliximab are options for the treatment of severe, active Crohn's disease, following inadequate response to conventional therapies or in those who are intolerant of or have contra-indications to conventional therapy. Vedolizumab is recommended for moderate

to severely active Crohn's disease when therapy with adalimumab or infliximab is unsuccessful, is contra-indicated or not tolerated. Ustekinumab is recommended for moderate to severely active Crohn's disease when conventional therapy or therapy with adalimumab or infliximab is unsuccessful, is contra-indicated or not tolerated.
https://bnfc.nice.org.uk/treatment-summaries/crohns-disease/

217 **C – Amoxicillin, metronidazole and lansoprazole for 7 days with no changes to the patient's regular medications.**
Clarithromycin is an inhibitor of the P-450 enzyme system which may potentiate the effect of amlodipine and atorvastatin. The interaction with atorvastatin can result in rhabdomyolysis and atorvastatin should be withheld during the course of treatment if clarithromycin is required. Clopidogrel is a pro-drug and omeprazole inhibits CYP2C19 enzyme, which converts clopidogrel to its active metabolite. Famotidine is a H2-receptor antagonist and not a proton pump inhibitor. Clarithromycin, metronidazole and lansoprazole is the first line combination for patients with penicillin allergy.
https://bnf.nice.org.uk/treatment-summaries/helicobacter-pylori-infection/

218 **C – Prednisolone**
Drugs that induce peptic ulcers include NSAIDs, aspirin, bisphosphonates, immunosuppressive agents (e.g. corticosteroids), potassium chloride, selective serotonin reuptake inhibitors (SSRIs). Clopidogrel can cause GI bleed, rather than peptic ulcers.
https://bnf.nice.org.uk/treatment-summaries/peptic-ulcer-disease/

219 **B – Enteric-coated tablet**
Enteric-coated and modified-release medicines are unsuitable in patients with an ileostomy, as there may be insufficient release of the active ingredient. Preparation forms with quick dissolution and absorption should be used - liquids, capsules, and uncoated or soluble tablets are usually well absorbed. When a solid-dose form such as a capsule or a tablet is given, the contents of the stoma bag should be checked for any remnants.
https://bnf.nice.org.uk/treatment-summaries/stoma-care/

220 D – Stop taking/using mesalazine immediately and see her GP as soon as possible

Patients receiving aminosalicylates and their carers should be advised to report any unexplained bleeding, bruising, purpura, sore throat, fever or malaise that occurs during treatment. These can be signs of agranulocytosis (especially if associated with a fever and rash) and treatment should be stopped immediately.

https://bnf.nice.org.uk/drugs/mesalazine/#patient-and-carer-advice

221 B – Monitor the need for therapy every 4-6 weeks until symptoms stabilise and then every 6-12 months

Therapy for urinary incontinence, in children should be monitored soon after it has been commenced and at regular intervals, and in adults every 4-6 weeks until symptoms are stable and then every 6-12 months.

https://bnf.nice.org.uk/drugs/oxybutynin-hydrochloride/#prescribing-and-dispensing-information

222 C – Lansoprazole

As per BNF - Hypomagnesaemia is listed as a side effect of proton pump inhibitors such as lansoprazole (more common after 1 year of treatment, but sometimes after 3 months of treatment). Measurement of serum-magnesium concentrations should be considered before and during prolonged treatment, especially when used with other drugs that cause hypomagnesaemia or with digoxin.

https://bnf.nice.org.uk/drugs/lansoprazole/

223 B – Long term NSAID use

Risk factors for the development of peptic ulcer include the use of drugs such as NSAIDs, aspirin, bisphosphonates, corticosteroids, potassium supplements and SSRIs.

https://cks.nice.org.uk/topics/dyspepsia-proven-peptic-ulcer/background-information/risk-factors/

224 D – Mebeverine

Antispasmodic drugs such as mebeverine, alverine or peppermint oil can be prescribed for IBS where there is ongoing abdominal pain or spasms.

https://cks.nice.org.uk/topics/irritable-bowel-syndrome/management/management/

Medium weighted answers | 153

225 B – Clindamycin
As per BNF – Diarrhoea is a common or very common side effect of clindamycin and treatment should be discontinued if this occurs.
https://bnf.nice.org.uk/drugs/clindamycin/

226 E – Take ONE 70mg tablet once a week
As per BNF – For female patients with postmenopausal osteoporosis the dose is 10mg daily or 70mg once weekly.
https://bnf.nice.org.uk/drugs/alendronic-acid/#indications-and-dose

227 E – Naproxen
NSAIDs such as naproxen are associated with serious gastro-intestinal toxicity; the risk is higher in the elderly.
https://bnf.nice.org.uk/drugs/naproxen/

228 C – Pain commences prior to the menstrual cycle
Dysmenorrhoea is characterised by painful cramping, usually in the lower abdomen, which usually occurs shortly before and/or during menstruation.
https://cks.nice.org.uk/topics/dysmenorrhoea/

229 C – Nitrofurantoin 100mg twice daily for 7 days
For pregnant women who have an uncomplicated urinary tract infection for the first time an immediate antibiotic such as cefalexin, amoxicillin of nitrofurantoin may be suitable treatment.
https://cks.nice.org.uk/topics/urinary-tract-infection-lower-women/management/uti-in-pregnancy-no-visible-haematuria/#management

230 E – Urine may turn yellow or brown
As per BNF – Discolouration of urine is listed as a side effect of nitrofurantoin – frequency not known.
https://bnf.nice.org.uk/drugs/nitrofurantoin/#side-effects

231 D – Lansoprazole
As per BNF – Lansoprazole is indicated for the prophylaxis of NSAID-associated duodenal ulcer and gastric ulcer.
https://bnf.nice.org.uk/drugs/lansoprazole/#indications-and-dose

232 B – Hyoscine butylbromide
As per BNF – Hyoscine butylbromide is indicated for the treatment of irritable bowel syndrome.
https://bnf.nice.org.uk/drugs/hyoscine-butylbromide/#indications-and-dose

233 G – Naloxegol
As per BNF – Naloxegol is licensed for opioid induced constipation when the response to other laxatives in inadequate.
https://bnf.nice.org.uk/drugs/naloxegol/#indications-and-dose

234 E – Mesalazine
As per BNF – Monitoring requirements for mesalazine are that renal function should be monitored before starting treatment, at 3 months, and then annually.
https://bnf.nice.org.uk/drugs/mesalazine/#monitoring-requirements

235 H – Ondansetron
As per BNF – Ondansetron is licensed for the treatment of nausea and vomiting in both cases of emetogenic chemotherapy or radiotherapy and postoperative nausea and vomiting.
https://bnf.nice.org.uk/drugs/ondansetron/#indications-and-dose

236 C – Ferrous sulphate
As per BNF - A diagnostic trial of oral iron treatment for 2-4 weeks may be considered in for pregnant women.
https://cks.nice.org.uk/topics/anaemia-iron-deficiency/diagnosis/diagnostic-trials-of-iron-treatment/

237 D – Folic acid
As per BNF – Folic acid is indicated for the treatment of folate-deficient megaloblastic anaemia and is continued until term in pregnant women.
https://bnf.nice.org.uk/drugs/folic-acid/#indications-and-dose

238 F – Thaimine
As per BNF - Parenteral thiamine, followed by oral thiamine, should be given to patients with suspected Wernicke's encephalopathy.
https://bnf.nice.org.uk/treatment-summaries/alcohol-dependence/

239 E – Hydroxocobalamin
As per BNF - Hydroxocobalamin is licensed for the treatment of pernicious anaemia and other macrocytic anaemias without neurological involvement at a dosage of initially 1 mg 3 times a week for 2 weeks, then 1 mg every 2–3 months.
https://bnf.nice.org.uk/drugs/hydroxocobalamin/

240 A – Colecalciferol
Colecalciferol is used as the treatment for vitamin D deficiency.
https://cks.nice.org.uk/topics/vitamin-d-deficiency-in-adults/

241 D – Methotrexate
As per BNF – Methotrexate is licensed for the treatment of both moderate and severe rheumatoid arthritis. In view of reports of blood dyscrasias (including fatalities) and liver cirrhosis with low-dose methotrexate patients should have full blood count and renal and liver function tests repeated every 1–2 weeks until therapy is stabilised and should be monitored every 2–3 months thereafter. Folic acid decreases mucosal and gastrointestinal side-effects of methotrexate and may prevent hepatotoxicity.
https://bnf.nice.org.uk/drugs/methotrexate/

242 H – Tacrolimus
As per BNF – Tacrolimus is licensed for the treatment of severe atopic eczema in patients who have not responded to conventional therapy.
https://bnf.nice.org.uk/drugs/tacrolimus/#indications-and-dose

243 E – Mycophenolate
As per BNF – Mycophenolate is licensed for the prevention of organ rejection following renal, hepatic and cardiac transplantation. This immunosuppressant medication is prescribed as prophylaxis to prevent organ rejection. It requires a full blood count every week for 4 weeks then twice a month for 2 months then every month in the first year (consider interrupting treatment if neutropenia develops).
https://bnf.nice.org.uk/drugs/mycophenolate-mofetil/#monitoring-requirements

244 E – Infliximab
As per BNF – Infliximab is licensed for the treatment of rheumatoid arthritis (in combination with methotrexate). Treatment is by infusion and under expert supervision.
https://bnf.nice.org.uk/drugs/infliximab/#indications-and-dose

245 A – Azathioprine
As per BNF – Azathioprine is licenced for severe Crohn's disease. It is metabolised to mercaptopurine. Blood tests and monitoring for signs of myelosuppression are essential in long-term treatment.
https://bnf.nice.org.uk/drugs/azathioprine/

246 D – Mirabegron
As per BNF – Mirabegron is licensed for the treatment of urinary frequency, urgency, and urge incontinence. Blood pressure should be monitored before starting treatment and regularly during treatment, especially in patients with pre-existing hypertension.
https://bnf.nice.org.uk/drugs/mirabegron/

247 G – Tamsulosin
As per BNF - Tamsulosin hydrochloride 400 microgram capsules can be sold to the public for the treatment of functional symptoms of benign prostatic hyperplasia in men aged 45–75 years to be taken for up to 6 weeks before clinical assessment by a doctor.
https://bnf.nice.org.uk/drugs/tamsulosin-hydrochloride/#exceptions-to-legal-category

248 C – Finasteride
As per BNF – Finasteride is licensed for the treatment of benign prostatic hyperplasia. It is excreted in semen and use of a condom is recommended if sexual partner is pregnant or likely to become pregnant.
https://bnf.nice.org.uk/drugs/finasteride/#conception-and-contraception

249 E – Oxybutynin
As per NICE CKS – Oxybutynin is used to treat lower urinary tract symptoms. It is an antimuscarinic and is available as a transdermal patch.
https://cks.nice.org.uk/topics/luts-in-men/prescribing-information/antimuscarinics/

250 H – Trimethoprim

As per BNF – Trimethoprim is licensed for the treatment of lower urinary tract infections.
https://bnf.nice.org.uk/drugs/trimethoprim/#indications-and-dose

251 C – Add montelukast and review in 6 weeks

As per NICE CKS – Monetelukast is a leukotriene receptor antagonist. NICE guidance is that if a patient's asthma is not adequately controlled with low-dose ICS alone, then consider a trial of an add-on therapy. For children (5 to 16 years) offer a leukotriene receptor antagonist (LTRA) in addition to the paediatric low dose ICS, and review the response in 4 to 8 weeks.
https://cks.nice.org.uk/topics/asthma/management/newly-diagnosed-asthma/

252 A – Beclometasone

As per NICE CKS – Beclometasone is an inhaled corticosteroid (ICS) and is used as preventer therapy for all people who use an inhaled SABA three times a week or more, and/or have asthma symptoms three times a week or more.
https://cks.nice.org.uk/topics/asthma/management/newly-diagnosed-asthma/

253 F – Salbutamol

As per BNF – High doses of salbutamol can cause akathisia and hypokalaemia.
https://bnf.nice.org.uk/drugs/salbutamol/#side-effects

254 E – Roflumilast

As per BNF - Roflumilast is a phosphodiesterase type-4 inhibitor with anti-inflammatory properties. It is licensed for the treatment of severe chronic obstructive pulmonary disease.
https://bnf.nice.org.uk/drugs/roflumilast/

255 H – Tiotropium

As per BNF – Tiotropium is licensed for the maintenance treatment of chronic obstructive pulmonary disease.
https://bnf.nice.org.uk/drugs/tiotropium/

256 G – Theophylline

As per BNF – Theophylline is licensed for the treatment of chronic asthma and requires dose adjustment may be required if smoking started or stopped during treatment.
https://bnf.nice.org.uk/drugs/theophylline/#indications-and-dose

Low weighted answers

257 A – Amitriptyline
Amitriptyline works by blocking muscarinic receptors from the action of acetylcholine. When these receptors are blocked, tear production stops, causing the eyes to be dry. Other common side effects caused by antimuscarinic drugs include dry mouth, constipation, urinary retention and blurred vision.
https://www.ncbi.nlm.nih.gov/books/ NBK537225/#:~:text=Amitriptyline%20is%20in%20the%20 tricyclic,to%20treat%20depression%20in%20adults.

258 D – Uveitis
Irregularly shaped pupils are a classic characteristic of uveitis.
https://cks.nice.org.uk/topics/uveitis/diagnosis/assessment/

259 A – Administer broad-spectrum antibacterial therapy according to local guidance
Cytotoxic drugs, such as melphalan, can cause bone marrow suppression. Peripheral blood counts must be checked before each treatment, and doses should be reduced or therapy delayed if bone-marrow has not recovered. Fever in a neutropenic patient (neutrophil count less than 1.06×10^9/litre) requires immediate broad-spectrum antibacterial therapy. Appropriate bacteriological investigations should be conducted as soon as possible. Patients taking cytotoxic drugs who have signs or symptoms of infection should be advised to seek prompt medical attention. All patients should initially be investigated and treated under the supervision of the appropriate oncology or haematology specialist.
https://bnf.nice.org.uk/treatment-summaries/cytotoxic-drugs/

260 **E – Vincristine**
When vinca alkaloids are injected intrathecally, destruction of the central nervous system occurs, radiating out from the injection site. If given intrathecally, vinca alkaloid is nearly always fatal and associated with an irreversible, painful ascending paralysis.
https://bnf.nice.org.uk/drugs/vincristine-sulfate-specialist-drug/

261 **D – Osteoporosis**
Osteoporosis is associated with androgen deprivation therapy. A bisphosphonate should be offered to patients who have osteoporosis and who are having androgen deprivation therapy; denosumab is an alternative if bisphosphonates are not appropriate. Enteropathy is often radiation-induced. Gynaecomastia can occur with long-term (longer than 6 months) bicalutamide treatment. Tumour flare due to an initial surge in testosterone concentrations has been reported in the initial stages of treatment with LHRH agonists. Cyproterone acetate, which is used to managed hot flushes associated with long term androgen suppression, can cause an increased risk of meningioma.
https://bnf.nice.org.uk/treatment-summaries/osteoporosis/

262 **A – Risk of cardiac failure**
Congestive heart failure (NYHA Class II to IV) is a common adverse reaction associated with the use of trastuzumab and has been associated with a fatal outcome. Cardiac function should be regularly assessed in patients receiving trastuzumab, and particular caution should be taken in patients with underlying cardiac disease.
https://bnf.nice.org.uk/drugs/trastuzumab-specialist-drug/#side-effects

263 **B – Letrozole**
In post-menopausal women with oestrogen-receptor positive invasive breast cancer who are at medium or high risk of disease recurrence, an aromatase inhibitor should be given as first line therapy. Alternatively, tamoxifen should be given if an aromatase inhibitor is not tolerated or is contra-indicated, or if the risk of disease recurrence is low. Trastuzumab is biological therapy and zoledronic acid is a bisphosphonate. Goserelin is a GnRH.
https://bnf.nice.org.uk/treatment-summaries/breast-cancer/ AND *https://bnf.nice.org.uk/drugs/letrozole/*

264 B – Colchicine

Acute attacks of gout are usually treated with colchicine, high dose NSAIDs (consider prescribing concurrent PPI) or a short course of oral corticosteroid. Colchicine is the most appropriate first line treatment for acute gout attack in this case. This patient has a background of asthma and NSAID use may trigger an acute asthma attack. Corticosteroids, such as prednisolone, may raise blood glucose level in patients with diabetes. Anakinra is an interleukin-1 inhibitor and should only be used for acute gout attack as last line under specialist advice.
https://bnf.nice.org.uk/treatment-summaries/gout/

265 B – 14-28 days after the flare

For long term control of gout, the formation of uric acid from purines may be reduced with xanthine-oxidase inhibitors (allopurinol or febuxostat). Treatment should be started at least 2-4 weeks after a gout flare has settled.
https://bnf.nice.org.uk/treatment-summaries/gout/

266 D – 360mmol/L

A treat-to-target strategy should be used when offering urate lowering therapy, this involves starting with a low dose of therapy and using monthly serum urate levels to guide dose increase, as tolerated, until the target serum urate level is reached. Aim for a target serum urate level below 360micromol/L.
https://bnf.nice.org.uk/treatment-summaries/gout/

267 A – Carbomer eye gel

Hypromellose is the most frequently used treatment for tear deficiency in patients with mild dry eye. Initially, it may need to be instilled frequently (e.g. hourly) for adequate symptom relief, then at a reduced frequency. Carbomers and polyvinyl alcohol are suitable alternatives. The ability of carbomers and polyvinyl alcohol to cling to the eye surface and their higher viscosity may help reduce frequency of application to 4 times daily. Carbomers can be less tolerated than hypromellose due to their impact on vision. Ocular lubricants containing sodium hyaluronate, hydroxypropyl guar, or carmellose sodium can be used for moderate to severe dry eye following a suitable trial (6–8 weeks) of treatment options for mild dry eye. Eye ointments containing a paraffin (e.g. liquid paraffin

with white soft paraffin and wool alcohols) can be used in addition to other options to lubricate the eye surface, especially in cases of recurrent corneal epithelial erosion. They may cause temporary visual disturbance and are best suited for application before sleep. Ointments should not be used during contact lens wear.
https://bnf.nice.org.uk/treatment-summaries/dry-eye/

268 **B – Bimatoprost**
Topical prostaglandin analogues include latanoprost, tafluprost, travoprost, or bimatoprost. Levobunolol hydrochloride is a topical beta-blocker. Dorzolamide is a carbonic anhydrase inhibitor. Apraclonidine and brimonidine tartrate are topical sympathomimetics.
https://cks.nice.org.uk/topics/glaucoma/prescribing-information/topical-prostaglandin-analogues-prostamides/

269 **C – 6 months**
Cimzia® (certolizumab pegol) is a tumour necrosis factor alpha (TFN-a) inhibitor. Following reports of death in neonates who received a live attenuated vaccine after exposure to a TNF-a inhibitor in utero, the MHRA has issued the following advice: An infant who has been exposed to TNF-a inhibitors and other immunosuppressive biological medicines in utero, PHE advise that any live attenuated vaccination (e.g. BCG vaccine) should be deferred until the infant is age 6 months.
https://bnf.nice.org.uk/drugs/certolizumab-pegol/

270 **C – 8 weeks**
Most eligible individuals should receive 2 doses of COVID-19 vaccine for their primary course; 3 doses are required for individuals aged 6 months and over who were severely immunosuppressed at the time of their vaccination. For most individuals, JCVI recommend a minimum 8-week interval between doses, unless rapid immunisation is required in specific circumstances (such as individuals about to receive immunosuppressive treatment). However, for healthy individuals aged under 18 years who are not health and social care workers, carers, or household contacts of immunosuppressed individuals, a minimum 12-week interval between doses is recommended.
https://bnf.nice.org.uk/treatment-summaries/covid-19-vaccines/#primary-immunisation

271 **E – Suxamethonium**
NMBAs are most commonly suspected to be triggers of perioperative anaphylactic reaction. Amongst the NMBAs, suxamethonium is almost twice as likely to cause anaphylaxis as other NMBAs, with a rate of 11.1 per 100,000 administrations.
https://bnf.nice.org.uk/drugs/suxamethonium-chloride/

272 **C – Inhibition of acetylcholine release**
Botulinum toxin is an exotoxin produced by the anaerobic bacterium *Clostridium botulinum* and can be used for therapeutic purposes. It inhibits acetylcholine release from nerve terminals.
https://bnf.nice.org.uk/drugs/botulinum-toxin-type-a/

273 **C – Fludrocortisone**
Two types of corticosteroids are mineralcorticoid and glucocorticoid. Mineralocorticoid effects are most marked with fludrocortisone acetate, but are also significant with hydrocortisone, corticotropin, and tetracosactide. Mineralocorticoid actions are negligible with the high potency glucocorticoids, betamethasone and dexamethasone, and occur only slightly with methylprednisolone, prednisolone, and triamcinolone.
https://bnf.nice.org.uk/treatment-summaries/corticosteroids-general-use/

274 **C – Mometasone furoate for 14 days**
In the management of acute sinusitis, children presenting with symptoms for around 10 days or less should be given advice about the usual duration of acute sinusitis, self-care of pain or fever with paracetamol or ibuprofen, and when to seek medical help. Children and their carers should be reassured that antibiotics are usually not required. Children (over the age of 12) presenting with symptoms for around 10 days or more with no improvement could be considered for treatment with a high-dose nasal corticosteroid, such as mometasone furoate (unlicensed use) or fluticasone (unlicensed use) for 14 days. If the child is systemically very unwell, has signs and symptoms of a more serious illness or condition, or is at high-risk of complications, an immediate antibiotic could be offered if deemed appropriate.
https://cks.nice.org.uk/topics/sinusitis/management/acute-sinusitis/

275 D – Offer OTC treatment with macrogol and advice on diet modification

The first-line treatment for children with constipation requires the use of a laxative in combination with dietary modification and behavioural interventions. Diet modification alone is not recommended as first-line treatment. If faecal impaction is not present (or has been treated), the child should be treated promptly with a laxative. A macrogol is preferred as first-line management, with the dose adjusted according to symptoms and response. If the response is inadequate add a stimulant laxative, or change to a stimulant laxative if the first-line therapy is not tolerated. If stools remain hard, lactulose or another laxative with softening effects, such as docusate, should be added.

https://bnf.nice.org.uk/treatment-summaries/constipation/#constipation-in-children

276 E – 2.5mg per hour infusion

The BNFc dose of glucagon for cardiogenic shock due to acute overdosage of beta-blockers is: 50–150 micrograms/kg (max. per dose 10 mg), administered over 1–2 minutes, followed by (by intravenous infusion) 50 micrograms/kg/hour, titrated according to response. The bolus dose (which has already been administered) is followed by an infusion at 50micrograms/kg/hour. The child is 50kg, so the infusion should start at 2.5mg (2500micrograms) per hour titrate according to response.

https://bnfc.nice.org.uk/drugs/glucagon/

277 D – 200mg.

As per BNFc - Child 7–9 years: 200 mg 3 times a day, maximum daily dose to be given in 3–4 divided doses; maximum 30 mg/kg per day; maximum 2.4 g per day. Note the child is 30kg so max dose is 900mg per day so option E is incorrect. Option A to C would be underdosing.

https://bnfc.nice.org.uk/drugs/ibuprofen/

278 C – As the patient is under 16-years-old, it is good practice for you to follow criteria set out in Fraser guidelines

In adolescents, hormonal contraception is used after menarche. When prescribing contraception for females aged under 16 years, it is considered good practice for health professionals to follow the criteria commonly known as the Fraser Guidelines. The Fraser guidelines apply specifically to advice and treatment about contraception and sexual health. They may be used by a range of healthcare professionals working with under 16-year-olds.

Gillick competency applies mainly to medical advice but it is also used by practitioners in other settings. Medical professionals need to consider Gillick competency if a young person under the age of 16 wishes to receive treatment without their parents' or carers' consent or, in some cases, knowledge.

https://www.fsrh.org/standards-and-guidance/documents/cec-ceu-guidance-young-people-mar-2010/

279 **A – Crotamiton is a suitable treatment to manage itching associated with scabies**
Permethrin and malathion are used for the treatment of scabies; malathion can be used if permethrin is inappropriate. Benzyl benzoate is an irritant and should be avoided in children; it is also less effective than malathion and permethrin. Although acaricides have traditionally been applied after a hot bath, this is not necessary and there is even evidence that a hot bath may increase absorption into the blood, removing them from their site of action on the skin. All members of the affected household should be treated simultaneously. Malathion and permethrin should be applied twice, one week apart; in the case of benzyl benzoate in adults, up to 3 applications on consecutive days may be needed.
https://cks.nice.org.uk/topics/scabies/management/management-of-scabies/

280 **C – The symptoms described could be a side effect of pioglitazone. The patient should stop taking pioglitazone immediately and arrange an appointment with the GP as soon as possible.**
There is a small increased risk of bladder cancer associated with pioglitazone use (MHRA/CHM advice) Pioglitazone should not be used in patients with active bladder cancer or a past history of bladder cancer, or in those who have uninvestigated macroscopic haematuria. Pioglitazone should be used with caution in elderly patients as the risk of bladder cancer increases with age. Before initiating treatment with pioglitazone, patients should be assessed for risk factors of bladder

cancer and any macroscopic haematuria should be investigated. The safety and efficacy of pioglitazone should be reviewed after 3–6 months and pioglitazone should be stopped in patients who do not respond adequately to treatment. Patients should be advised to report promptly any haematuria, dysuria, or urinary urgency during treatment.
https://bnf.nice.org.uk/drugs/pioglitazone/#important-safety-information

281 **D – Pre-treatment monitoring of sodium valproate include liver function test and full blood count**
Sodium valproate in licensed in the treatment of epilepsy, mania but not licensed for the prophylaxis of migraine. In the treatment of epilepsy, Sodium Valproate is a Category 2 drug - the need for continued supply of a particular manufacturer's product should be based on clinical judgement and consultation with the patient and/or carer taking into account factors such as seizure frequency, treatment history, and potential implications to the patient of having a breakthrough seizure. Sodium valproate is tetarogenic, the MHRA advises that all women and girls of childbearing potential being treated with valproate medicines must be supported on a Pregnancy Prevention Programme—pregnancy should be excluded before treatment initiation and highly effective contraception must be used during treatment. If sodium valproate is stopped, abrupt withdrawal should be avoided; the dose should be gradually reduced over at least 4 weeks.
https://bnf.nice.org.uk/drugs/sodium-valproate/

282 **E – Pharmacy professionals must speak up when they have concerns or when things go wrong**
Note the question asks for best-demonstrated GPhC standard. Duty of candour is not a GPhC standard (although there is a GPhC guidance available for this). Pharmacy professionals must speak up when they have concerns or when things go wrong:

At the heart of this standard is the requirement to be candid with the person concerned and with colleagues and employers. This is usually called the 'duty of candour' – which means being honest when things go wrong. People receive safe and effective care when pharmacy professionals
- are open and honest when things go wrong
- say sorry, provide an explanation and put things right when things go wrong

- reflect on feedback or concerns, taking action as appropriate and thinking about what can
- be done to prevent the same thing happening again
- improve the quality of care and pharmacy practice by learning from feedback and when things go wrong

https://www.pharmacyregulation.org/pharmacists/standards-and-guidance-pharmacy-professionals/standards-pharmacy-professionals

283 B – MHRA

The MHRA monitors new medicines intensively to ensure that any new safety hazards are identified promptly. The Commission on Human Medicines (CHM) and the MHRA encourages the reporting of all suspected reactions to newer drugs and vaccines, which are denoted by an inverted black triangle symbol (▼). This symbol appears next to the name of a relevant product in: a drug safety update; the BNF and NPF; the monthly index of medical specialities (MIMS); and advertising material. The MHRA assesses the Black Triangle status of a product usually 2 years after marketing; however, there is no standard time for a product to retain Black Triangle status.

https://www.gov.uk/drug-safety-update/the-black-triangle-scheme-or

284 E – Schedule 4 Part 1 CD

Lorazepam

https://bnf.nice.org.uk/drugs/lorazepam/medicinal-forms/#oral-tablet
AND *MEP – Classification of medicines*

285 C – Rifaximin

As per BNF – Rifaximin is cautioned for discolouring soft contact lenses.
https://bnf.nice.org.uk/drugs/rifampicin/#cautions

286 C – Advise him to contact his GP today

The most important side-effect of the penicillins is hypersensitivity which causes rashes and anaphylaxis and can be fatal. Allergic reactions to penicillins occur in 1–10% of exposed individuals; anaphylactic reactions occur in fewer than 0.05% of treated patients.

https://bnf.nice.org.uk/drugs/phenoxymethylpenicillin/#patient-and-carer-advice

287 E – 28 days
Tramadol is a schedule 3 CD. The maximum validity for schedule 3 CD prescriptions is 28 days.
MEP – Controlled drugs - Classification

288 B – 72 hours
For EEA prescribers you should follow the usual emergency supply process. Where the request originates from an approved health professional then a prescription needs to be received within 72 hours.
MEP - Prescriptions from the EEA or Switzerland

289 H – 6 months
Due to its low strength morphine sulfate 10mg/5ml is a schedule 5 CD. The maximum validity for schedule 5 CD is 6 months.
MEP – Controlled drugs - Classification

290 E – 28 days
Pregabalin is a schedule 3 CD. The maximum validity for schedule 3 CD prescriptions is 28 days.
MEP – Controlled drugs - Classification

291 F – 30 days
In cases of a request from a patient, if the emergency supply is for a CD the maximum quantity that can be supplied is for five days' treatment. For any other POM, no more than 30 days can be supplied.
MEP - Exemptions: sale and supply without a prescription

292 D – Under the PPP, prescriptions are only valid for 7 days
Under the PPP, prescriptions for oral retinoids are valid for 7 days only.
MEP – Pregnancy prevention programmes

293 E – The name and address of the prescribing veterinary surgeon must appear on the dispensing label
Only the name of the prescribing veterinary surgeon is required to appear on the label.
MEP - Labelling of dispensed veterinary medicines

294 C – Processing waste stock medicines or patient returned medicines
The pharmacist must be signed in but physical supervision is not required.
MEP – The responsible pharmacist

295 A – Information on the nature of the emergency
Information on the nature of the emergency only needs to be included in the pom register entry when the emergency supply is at the request of the patient.
MEP - Signed orders and record keeping

296 E – Oxycodone for injection
Physiotherapist independent prescribers can only prescribe oral oxycodone.
MEP – Prescriber types and prescribing restrictions

297 E – Treatment should not exceed 9 months
As per SPC – treatment should not exceed six months.
https://www.medicines.org.uk/emc/product/6533/smpc

298 C – Daktacort® hydrocortisone cream
All the OTC products listed are used to treat athletes foot, however Daktacort® hydrocortisone contains a steroid which would help relieve the patients itch.
https://bnf.nice.org.uk/treatment-summaries/topical-corticosteroids/

299 A – Refer to GP
People with diabetes should not use OTC products to treat warts or verrucae without advice from a nurse or doctor since impaired circulation, if present, can lead to delayed healing, ulceration or even gangrene.
https://bnf.nice.org.uk/drugs/salicylic-acid/

300 A – A history of five migraine attacks occurring over a period of one year
Sumatriptan can be supplied over-the-counter for those with a history of five or more attacks occurring over a period of one year – the migraine must be diagnosed by a doctor or pharmacist. All other cases in the question are contraindicated with the use of OTC sumatriptan.
https://www.rpharms.com/resources/pharmacy-guides/sumatriptan-p-medicine

301 A – Nurofen® plus
Nurofen® plus contains ibuprofen – this product is not licensed for use in asthmatics as ibuprofen can trigger symptoms of asthma or allergy.
https://www.medicines.org.uk/emc/product/5627

302 D – 240mg
The dose of paracetamol syrup 120mg/5ml for children 4 to 6 years is 10ml every 6 hours. 10ml is 240mg.
https://www.medicines.org.uk/emc/files/pil.6634.pdf

303 C – Paracetamol or ibuprofen can be used to reduce fever or pain
Ibuprofen should not be used to reduce fever or pain associated with chickenpox as it can cause more serious infections such as necrotising fasciitis.
Chickenpox - NHS (www.nhs.uk)

304 B – Impetigo
Impetigo presents as a red itchy sore. These break open and leak pus. As they heal, a crusty yellow scab starts to form. It is very common to see this around the mouth, especially in young children
https://www.lohiderm.com/articles/aad_education_library/920177-impetigo

305 A – Aching fingers, wrists or knees
Aching of the fingers, wrists or knees is more commonly associated with rubella.
https://cks.nice.org.uk/topics/scarlet-fever/ AND https://cks.nice.org.uk/topics/rubella/

306 E – work independently
As per MEP - Standard 2.
MEP - Appendix 1 - A Competency Framework for all Prescribers

307 C – Maintain, develop and use their professional knowledge and skills
As per MEP - Standard 4.
MEP - Appendix 1- A Competency Framework for all Prescribers

308 E – Pharmacy professionals recognise their own values and beliefs but do not impose them on other people
As per MEP - Standard 1.
MEP - Appendix 1- A Competency Framework for all Prescribers

309 D – Respect and maintain the person's confidentiality and privacy
As per MEP - Standard 7.
MEP - Appendix 1- A Competency Framework for all Prescribers

310 D – Pneumococcal vaccine
Individuals with an absent or dysfunctional spleen are at increased risk of severe infection, particularly those caused by encapsulated bacteria. The commonest organism associated with severe infection in these patients is the pneumococcus (Streptococcus pneumoniae).
https://assets.publishing.service.gov.uk/media/5e18a52940f0b65dc1918763/Greenbook_chapter_7_Immunsing_immunosupressed.pdf

311 A – Azithromycin 1 g once daily for 1 day
As per SPC - In uncomplicated chlamydia trachomatis urethritis and cervicitis the dose is 1,000 mg as a single oral dose.
https://www.medicines.org.uk/emc/product/6541/smpc

312 A – BCG vaccine
Mainly given to babies and young children who are at higher risk of getting TB, the BCG (Bacillus Calmette-Guérin) vaccine helps protect against tuberculosis.
https://www.nhs.uk/vaccinations/bcg-vaccine-for-tuberculosis-tb/

313 D – 180 mg every 4–6 hours; maximum 4 doses per day
OTC dosing – 2-4 years 7.5 ml (180 mg) Up to 4 times in 24 hours
https://www.medicines.org.uk/emc/files/pil.6634.pdf

314 A – Consider switching treatment to a patch
Refer the patient due to poor compliance.
https://bnf.nice.org.uk/treatment-summaries/contraceptives-hormonal/

Low weighted answers | 171

315 **F – Subconjunctival haemorrhage**
Red eye, when not accompanied with red flag signs, can be managed in primary care. The haemorrhage will clear in 1–2 weeks.
https://cks.nice.org.uk/topics/red-eye/management/management-of-red-eye/

316 **C – Dry eye**
Dry eye usually affects patients bilaterally. Symptoms include: eye irritation, itching, or discomfort; eye dryness (not always present); transient blurring of vision; watery eyes; redness of the eyelids or conjunctiva; photosensitivity; mucous discharge; eye fatigue; and contact lens intolerance. Management includes tear substitutes if lifestyle measures do not provide relief.
https://cks.nice.org.uk/topics/dry-eye-disease/

317 **B – Blepharitis**
Blepharitis usually affects both eyes, and is usually worse on a morning. It is a chronic, intermittent condition that can usually be controlled with self-care measures such as eyelid hygiene and warm compresses. If self-care measures are ineffective then topical or oral antibiotics can be prescribed.
https://cks.nice.org.uk/topics/blepharitis/

318 **A – Bacterial conjunctivitis**
Bacterial conjunctivitis is characterised by unilateral purulent discharge with crusting of the lids, that may be stuck together on waking. It is self-limiting but can be treated with over-the-counter topical antibiotics.
https://cks.nice.org.uk/topics/conjunctivitis-infective/

319 **H – Refer to A&E**
Symptoms suggest this could be a peritonsillar abscess/quinsy which requires immediate medical attention.
https://cks.nice.org.uk/topics/sore-throat-acute/

320 **C – Benzydamine oral spray**
Symptoms suggest sore throat. The condition usually clears up in a week. Benzydamine is a NSAID that reduces pain and inflammation.
https://cks.nice.org.uk/topics/sore-throat-acute/

321 E – Olive oil ear drops

Symptoms of impacted earwax include: hearing loss (most common symptom); blocked ears; ear discomfort; feeling of fullness in the ear; earache; tinnitus; itchiness; vertigo and cough (rare). Olive oil drops will soften wax and aid removal. Advise the person to use the drops 3–4 times daily for 3–5 days initially.

https://cks.nice.org.uk/topics/earwax/

322 G – Permethrin 5% cream

For scabies apply permethrin 5% cream over whole body including face, neck, scalp and ears then wash off after 8–12 hours. Treatment should be applied once weekly for 2 weeks.

https://bnf.nice.org.uk/drugs/permethrin/#indications-and-dose

323 D – Hydrocortisone 1% cream

Skin creams and ointments containing hydrocortisone (alone or with other ingredients) can be sold to the public for the treatment of allergic contact dermatitis, irritant dermatitis, insect bite reactions and mild to moderate eczema in patients over 10 years, to be applied sparingly over the affected area 1–2 times daily for a maximum period of a week.

https://bnf.nice.org.uk/drugs/hydrocortisone/#exceptions-to-legal-category

324 E – Ketoconazole 2% shampoo

Seborrhoeic dermatitis is associated with species of the yeast *Malassezia* and affects the scalp, paranasal areas, and eyebrows. Shampoos active against the yeast including those containing ketoconazole are used.

https://bnf.nice.org.uk/treatment-summaries/eczema/

325 A – Clobetasone butyrate 0.05% cream

Clobetasone butyrate 0.05% cream is listed as a moderate potency steroid based cream. The potency of all topical corticosteroids should be included on the label with the directions for use.

https://bnf.nice.org.uk/drugs/clobetasone-butyrate/#indications-and-dose

326 F – Mometasone furoate 1% cream

Mometasone furoate 1% cream is listed as a potent steroid based cream. As above, potency is a labelling requirement for all topical corticosteroids.

https://bnf.nice.org.uk/drugs/mometasone-furoate/

327 D – Sell chloramphenicol 0.5% eye drops

Bacterial conjunctivitis may be associated with purulent or mucopurulent discharge with crusting of the lids which may be stuck together on waking, as well as discomfort which may be described as 'grittiness', a 'foreign body' or 'burning' sensation. Conjunctivitis is characterised and associated with a yellow sticky discharge with symptoms being described as gritty rather than painful. Although this is self-limiting, the patient states they are going to a party so would prefer treatment. Chloramphenicol eye drops can be sold in pharmacies and are suitable for adults and children over the age of 2 years. Due to their age, you can sell this at the patient's request.

https://cks.nice.org.uk/topics/conjunctivitis-infective/diagnosis/clinical-features/ AND *https://cks.nice.org.uk/topics/conjunctivitis-infective/management/management-in-primary-care/*

328 C – Store in a refrigerator between 2-8°C and discard after 28 days from opening

As per SPC - Special precautions for storage: protect from light; store in a refrigerator at a temperature between 2°C and 8°C; discard remaining contents 28 days after opening.

https://www.medicines.org.uk/emc/product/427/smpc#gref

329 E – Zovirax® cream (aciclovir 5% cream)

Aciclovir cream is the most appropriate medication to suggest as it can treat herpes simplex and reduce the time taken for the lesion to heal. Blistex®, Carmex® and petroleum jelly are all used as a moisturiser for lips. Bonjela® is used to manage mouth ulcers. Zovirax® is licensed to manage herpes simplex.

https://bnf.nice.org.uk/drugs/aciclovir/#indications-and-dose

330 B – Dry gritty eyes

Patients with sepsis will not usually have dry gritty eyes- all the other symptoms can be seen in sepsis.

https://cks.nice.org.uk/topics/sepsis/ AND
https://www.nhs.uk/conditions/sepsis/

331 B – Refer to GP
The patient needs to be referred to GP as the eczema on their hands is infected- they are cracked and weeping. Topical hydrocortisone should not be sold for application to the face, anogenital region, and broken or infected skin.
https://bnf.nice.org.uk/drugs/hydrocortisone/#exceptions-to-legal-category

332 A – It is strongly recommended that all members of the family are treated at the same time
Care should be taken to avoid re-infection and it is strongly recommended that all members of the family are treated at the same time.
https://www.medicines.org.uk/emc/product/75/smpc#gref AND https://www.nhs.uk/conditions/threadworms/#:~:text=You%20can%20buy%20medicine%20(mebendazole,you're%20pregnant%20or%20breastfeeding.

333 F – 18 years
This medicine can be taken by adults between the ages of 18 and 65 years.
https://www.medicines.org.uk/emc/files/pil.8337.pdf

334 C – 10 years
Topical hydrocortisone preparations can be supplied to patients OTC over the age of 10 years.
https://bnf.nice.org.uk/drugs/hydrocortisone/#exceptions-to-legal-category

335 E – 16 years
Fluconazole capsules can be sold to the public, aged 16–60 years, for treament of vaginal candidiasis and associated candidal balanitis.
https://bnf.nice.org.uk/drugs/fluconazole/#exceptions-to-legal-category

336 D – 12 years
The dosage for adults and children over 12 years is 1 tablet every 4 to 6 hours up to 4 times a day.
https://www.medicines.org.uk/emc/product/6199/smpc

337 F – 18 years
Due to the lack of clinical data, amorolfine 5% w/v medicated nail lacquer is not recommended for patients below the age of 18 years.
https://www.medicines.org.uk/emc/product/7414/smpc

338 A – 4 months
Miconazole gel is indicated for the oral treatment of superficial fungal infections of the oropharynx in adults and paediatric patients 4 months and older.
https://www.medicines.org.uk/emc/product/6597/smpc

339 B – 2 years
Mebendazole can be used in the treatment of threadworm in adults and children over the age of 2 years.
https://www.medicines.org.uk/emc/product/1317/smpc

340 G – 45 years
Tamsulosin hydrochloride 400 microgram capsules can be sold to the public for the treatment of functional symptoms of benign prostatic hyperplasia in men aged 45–75.
https://bnf.nice.org.uk/drugs/tamsulosin-hydrochloride/

341 E – 16 years
2% external clotrimazole cream and 500mg clotrimazole pessary cannot be used by children below 16 years.
https://www.medicines.org.uk/emc/product/5532/smpc

Calculations answers

342 C – 1200mg/L
5 hrs – 3000mg/L;
10 hrs – 1500mg/L;
15 hrs – 750mg/L;
12 hrs 1200 mg/L

343 B – 90
Day 1 – 5 = 60mg × 5 = 300mg;
Day 6 = 50mg;
Day 7 = 40mg;
Day 8 = 30mg;
Day 9 = 20mg;
Day 10 = 10mg.

300 + 50 + 40 + 30 + 20 + 10 = 450
450 ÷ 5 = 90

344 £885
Calculate the cost for 1 patient on original treatment:
Nitrofurantoin 100mg capsules – 1 twice a day for five days, need 10 capsules to complete treatment.
Calculate cost of 10 capsules:
   (£9.75 ÷ 14) × 10 = £6.96 per patient

Calculate cost of for 1 patient on new proposed treatment:
Nitrofurantoin 100mg tablets – 1 twice a day for five days, need 10 tablets for the treatment.
Calculate cost for 10 tablets (£3.00 ÷ 28) × 10= £1.07 per patient
Calculate the total saved per patient:
   £6.96 – 1.04 = £5.89

Calculate total for 150 patients:
  £5.89 × 150 = £883.50 to the nearest £5 is £885.
Alternate working:
Calculate costs for 1500 caps (10 caps for 150 patients) and 1500 tablets and calculate the difference.

345 975 micrograms/min
Calculate the dose the patient takes during the infusion:
  78 × 0.75mg = 58.5mg over 60 minutes
Calculate the rate per minute:
  58.5 ÷ 6 0 = 0.975mg per minute
Convert to micrograms:
  0.975 × 1000 = 975 micrograms

346 349.42g
Calculate the total weight of the suppositories:
  175 × 2g = 350g
Total weight of drug:
  5mg × 175 = 875mg = 0.875g
Calculate the DV:
  Weight of drug in grams that displaces 1g of suppository base
  DV of diazepam is 1.5 therefore 0.875g of diazepam displaces 0.5833332g of base.
Calculate total base left:
  350 − 0.5833332g = 349.41667g,
  rounded to to 2 decimal places = 349.42g.

347 4800mg
Calculate how much estradiol needed in 100 g: 0.8% means 0.8g of drug in 100 g of base, 0.8 ÷ 100 × 600 = 4.8 g of estradiol needed.
Convert to milligrams: 4.8 × 1000 = 4800 mg.

348 932mg
Calculate the number of vials needed to cover treatment: 3 vials per day for 5 days= 15 vials.
Work out total amount of Na+:
  Each vial contains 2.7mmol, 2.7 × 15 = 40.5mmol

1 mole = 23 g; 1 mmol = 23 mg; 40.5 mmol = 931.5 mg.
932 mg to the nearest whole number.

349 10 hours

Start with the initial drug levels and then consider strength after each half-life

1280 → 640 → 32 0→ 160 → 80 → 40 → 20

It took 6 half-lives for the drug to reach 20 micrograms/mL which is 60 hours

One half-life is 60 ÷ 6 = 10.

350 £2830

Calculate amount of liquid used for 90 days:

dose 5mL daily × 90 = 450mL.

Calculate cost for 450 mL:

50.60 ÷ 150 × 450 = £151.80 COST for solution ONE patient for 90 days (or can calculate as 150ml x 3 needed so £50.60 × 3= £151.80)

Calculate cost for 90 tablets:

0.92 ÷ 28 × 90 = £2.96 COST FOR TABS for ONE patient

Total saved for one person for 90 days = £148.84

Multiply by 19 patients:

19 × 148.84 = £2827.96, rounded to the nearest £10 = £2830.

351 215mL

Calculate dose of capsules over 9 days:

Day 1:12 capsules,
Day 2: 8 capsules,
Day 3: 6 capsules,
Day 4, 5, 6: 12 capsules,
Day 7 &8: 4 capsules,
Day 9: 1 capsule.
Total 43 capsules.

Calculate equivalent dose in solution: 192mg capsule is equivalent to 157.7mg oral solution. Therefore 157.7/ 31.54 = 5mL, each capsule is equivalent to 5mL.

43 capsules × 5mL = 215mL to cover course.

352 14.58mL/hr

Calculate dose for 24hour infusion:

50mcg × 70 = 3500 mcg over 24 hours = 3.5mg over 24 hours.

Calculate how much 0.001% solution is needed: 0.001% is 0.001g per 100mL. This is the same as 1mg per 100mL. Which is the same as 3.5mg in 350mL. 350mL is administered over 24 hours.

350 ÷ 24 = 14.583333 mL/hr, round to 2 decimal places = 14.58mL/hr.

353 28.89% w/v

Calculate in parts what you have:

1750mL of 20% (remember 250mL discarded)

20g per 100mL so 350g in 1750mL

500mL of 60%

60g per 100mL so in 300g in 500mL

Total is 650g in 2250mL

28.888g per 100mL

So 28.89% w/v to 2 decimal places.

354 32 hours

Calculate how many half-lives to reduce from 400 mcg/litre

400 → 200 → 100 → 50 → 25

This takes 4 half lives

Each half-life is 8 hours so 4 × 8 = 32 hours.

355 112 tablets

Calculate the dose for the patient:

43 kg × 3mg = 129mg of ferrous iron daily.

If each 200mg tablet is the equivalent of 65mg of iron salt:

129mg ÷ 65mg = 1.9846 tablets daily

This is not practical so needs to take 2 tablets daily.

Total for 56 days: 56 × 2 = 112 tablets.

356 12 packs

Draw a table with the reducing dose

Dose in mg	Number of tablets	Days taken for	Total tablets	Cumulative total
45	9	7	63	63
40	8	7	56	119
35	7	7	49	168
30	6	7	42	210
25	5	7	35	245
20	4	7	28	273
15	3	7	21	294
10	2	7	14	308
5	1	28	28	336

Total 336 tablets

$336 \div 28 = 12$ packs.

357 48.8mL

Calculate dose of lidocaine needed:

4 mg/kg $= 61 \times 4 = 244$ mg needed

Calculate amount of lidocaine 0.5 % needed:

0.5 % means 0.5 g in 100 mL which is 500 mg in 100 mL. 5mg per mL.

Total for 244mg:

$244 \div 5 = 48.8$ mL.

Alternate working is:

$(244 \div 500) \times 100 = 48.8$ mL.

358 3mL

Calculate how many mg per mL:

100mg in 5mL therefore 20mg in 1mL. Hence 10mg in 0.5mL.

Calculate how many mL per 60mg:

0.5mL $\times 6 = 60$mg in 3mL.

359 10.5g

Calculate daily dose:

Each day the patient takes 3×500mg $= 1500$mg amoxicillin

Calculate total for 7 days:

7×1500mg $= 10500$mg

Convert mg to g: 10500mg $\div 1000 = 10.5$g.

Calculations answers | 181

360 97%

Calculate the total amount of sodium taken daily:
Each tablet contains 388 mg of sodium
388mg × 6 tablets = 2328mg = 2.328g per day
Calculate the daily dose as a percentage of daily allowance of sodium:
100% daily allowance = 2.4g of sodium each day.
2.328 ÷ 2.4 × 100 = 97%.

361 3.78g

Calculate estimated creatinine clearance using the formula provided:
(Constant = 1.23 for men)

$$\text{Estimated creatinine clearance in mL/min} = \frac{(140 - 62) \times 63 \times 1.23}{250}$$

$$= 24.17688 \text{ mL/min}$$

Read off dose adjustment from table and calculate:
Therefore patient needs to take
20mg/kg every 8 hours = 20 mg × 63 kg = 1260mg every 8 hours
Total over 24 hours = 1260mg × 3 = 3780 mg daily dose.
Convert into grams: 3.78g in 24 hours.

362 19.6mL

The displacement value is 0.4 mL/ 600 mg.
To get 600 mg at a final concentration of 30 mg/mL = 600 ÷ 30 = 20mL
The total volume needs to be 20 mL - so need to minus 0.4mL as this is displaced by 600mg of drug
Hence 19.6 mL of water for injection is needed to reconstitute each single vial.

363 8 hours

Calculate estimated creatinine clearance using the formula provided:
(Constant = 1.23 for men)

$$\text{Estimated creatinine clearance in mL/min} = \frac{(140 - 61) \times 46 \times 1.23}{120}$$

$$= 37.2485 \text{mL/min}$$

CrCl is 37.25mL/min therefore doses should be given every 8 hours according to the table above.

364 4.75% w/v

The new drug is used as a mouthwash at a concentration of 0.475% w/v. If this has been made from a solution that has been diluted 1 in 10, multiplying by 10 will give you the concentration of the intermediate solution. $0.475 \times 10 = 4.75\%$ no need to round as answer is to 2 decimal places.

365 48mL/min

The patient has congestive heart failure so need to use the following formula:

Digoxin clearance (mL/minute) =
  $(0.33 \times$ weight in kg$) + (0.9 \times$ creatinine clearance mL/minute$)$
  $(0.33 \times 69$ kg$) + (0.9 \times 28)$ mL/minute $= 22.77 + 25.2 = 47.97$

Need to round to nearest whole number = 48mL/min.

366 123mg

Read this question carefully, key points to highlight:
- The patient is coming in for her first etoposide infusion.
- She is to receive the same dose for five consecutive days.
- Maximum dosing is required.
- The patient's creatinine clearance is provided at 37mL/min

For dosing information, see section 4.2 Posology and method of administration in the SmPC provided. Under adult population, you will find the following information:

The recommended dose of etoposide in adult patients is 50-100 mg/m2 /day on days 1 to 5 or 100 to 120 mg/ m2 on days 1, 3, and 5 every 3 to 4 weeks in combination with other drugs indicated in the disease to be treated. Dosage should be modified to consider the myelosuppressive effects of other drugs in the combination or the effects of prior radiotherapy or chemotherapy (see section 4.4) which may have compromised bone marrow reserve.

The doses after the initial dose should be adjusted if neutrophil count is below 500 cells/mm3 for more than 5 days. In addition, the dose should be adjusted in case of occurrence of fever, infections, or at a thrombocyte count below 25,000 cells/mm3, which is not caused by the disease.

Follow up doses should be adjusted in case of occurrence of grade 3 or 4 toxicities or if renal creatinine clearance is below 50 ml/min.

At decreased creatinine clearance of 15 to 50 mL/min a dose reduction by 25% is recommended

Due to this, we know the dose is 100mg/m2 on day 1 – this is the dose if taking for 5 consecutive days.

$$\text{Patient BSA is } \sqrt{\frac{(156 \times 62)}{3600}} = 1.6391054 \text{ m}^2$$

Using BSA can calculate the dose needed:

1.6391054 m² × 100mg = 163.91054 mg of etoposide received. However, we have been given the information that:

At decreased creatinine clearance of 15 to 50 ml/min a dose reduction by 25% is recommended.

So calculated dose needs reduction:

163.91054 × 0.75 = 122.9329mg

123mg to nearest whole number.

367 1.7mL/min

From the extract we know we must administer 2g for each infusion and we must administer 40mg/mL over 30 mins. 2g is 2000mg, if we are to achieve a concentration of 40mg per mL, this means there is a total of 2 g in 50ml which is then given over 30 minutes.

50mL ÷ 30 minutes = 1.66666mL/min.

To 1 decimal place 1.7mL/min.

368 12 vials

Do ensure you are using correct units - BSA is calculated using height in centimetres.

$$BSA = \sqrt{\frac{(\text{height (cm)} \times \text{weight (kg)})}{3600}}$$

Using the formula given, BSA = 1.66 m

Dose = 1.66m² × 10mg = 16.6mg = 4 vials/day (available as 5 mg vials)
4 vials × 3 days = 12 vials.

369 0.9mg
0.15(L/Kg) × 68kg = 10.2L
10.2L × 80mcg = 816 mcg
Bioavailability of IV is 100%, therefore F = 1 × 0.88 = 0.88
816 ÷ 0.88 = 927.27mcg
loading dose = 927.27 mcg = 0.92 mg = 0.9mg.

370 0.14L
$C_1 \times V_1 = C_2 \times V_2$
1 in 4000 = 0.025% w/v (C2)
  (side note: 1% w/v = 1g/100mL in percentage weight by volume)
0.025 × 30 (dilution factor) = 0.75 (C1)
150 mL × 2 × 5 days = 4200 mL (V2)

$C_1 \times V_1 = C_2 \times V_2$
0.75 × ? = 0.025 × 4,200
? = 105 ÷ 0.75 = 140mL = 0.14L.

371 166.7mL
$C_1 \times V_1 = C_2 \times V_2$
4% (used at concentration) × 5 (dilution factor) = 20% (C2)
30 × ? = 20 × 500 (rearranged: (20 x 500) ÷ 30 = V_1
V_1 = 333.33mL (volume of stock solution)
500mL − 333.33mL = 166.67mL = 166.7mL.

372 6g
30 × 20/100 = 6 (surplus)
Total suppository is 36
36 × 200mg = 7,200mg = 7.2g
36 × 50mg = 1800mg = 1.8g
DV of 1.5 means 1.5g of drug displaces 1g of theobroma oil base
Therefore 1.8 grams of drug must displace 1.2 grams of base
7.2g − 1.2g = 6g.

373 2.7 mL

A 100mg/mL solution contains 100mg in 1mL, or 300mg in 3mL
The final volume required must therefore be 3mL
600 mg sodium valproate displaces 0.6mL, so 300mg must displace 0.3mL
3mL − 0.3mL = 2.7mL (volume of solvent required).

374 £2,220

30 × 90/100 = 27 patients eligible
Saving per patient per 30-day period: £43.12 − £15.73 = £27.39
Saving over 3 repeats per patient: £27.39 × 3 = £82.17
Saving for total number patients:
  £82.17 × 27 = £2,218.59 = £2,220 (nearest £10).

375 20

ARI = EER - CER
7.5% - 2.5% = 5% (ARI)
100%/5% OR 1/0.05 = 20 (which means for every 20 patients treated 1 patient will be harmed).

376 80 tablets

Longest duration of medication will last 27 days
28 tabs of metformin will last 7 days at current dose of 4 tablets daily, meaning 20 days quantity required
  20 × 4 = 80 tabs.

377 112 tablets

40mg daily = 8 tabs (8 × 5mg):
8 tabs × 3 = 24 tabs;
7 tabs × 3 = 21 tabs;
6 tabs × 3 = 18 tabs;
5 tabs × 3 = 15 tabs;
4 tabs × 3 = 12 tabs;
3 tabs × 3 = 9 tabs;
2 tabs × 3 = 6 tabs;
1 tabs × 7 = 7 tabs
  Total = 112 tabs.

378 1.8mL
Day 1 (prior) = 4 drops;
Day 2 (surgery day) = 4 drops;
2 weeks post-surgery = 4 × 14 = 56 drops.
Total 64 drops
64 ÷ 20 = 3.2mL used
5mL − 3.2mL = 1.8mL.

379 4mL
15mg in 10mL = 1.5mg in 1mL
6 ÷ 1.5 = 4mL daily.

380 166 mins
0.8mL × 40kg = 32mL ÷ 60 × 30 = 16mL ⎫
1.2mL × 40kg = 48mL ÷ 60 × 40 = 32mL ⎬ Total: 108mL
1.8mL × 40kg = 72mL ÷ 60 × 50 = 60mL ⎭
0.8g × 40 = 32g
16% (16g/100mL) = 32g/200mL (total volume infused)
200mL − 108mL = 92mL
3mL × 40kg ÷ 60mins = 2mL/min
92mL ÷ 2mL = 46min
46 + 30 + 40 + 50 minutes = 166 minutes.

381 0.48 mL/min
38kg × 50mg = 1,900mg / 2 (divided doses) = 950mg
Available as 500mg/5mL
950mg ÷ 500mg × 5mL = 9.5mL
9.5mL ÷ 20min = 0.475L/min.
Rounded to 2 decimal places = 0.48mL/min.

382 93.6%
1mmol = 58.5mg (Moles = Mass/Mr)
12mmol = 702mg (1 sachet)
8 (sachets) = 5,616mg = 5.616g
5616mg/6000mg (daily intake) (or 5.616g/6g) × 100 = 93.6%.

383 8.9 g

40 mmol/500 mL = 120 mmol/1,500 mL
1 mol = 74.5 g;
1 mmol = 74.5 mg;
120 mmol = 8940 mg;
8940 mg = 8.94 g = 8.9 g.

384 75mL/min

Using the formula provided (Constant = 1.23 for men)

$$\text{Estimated creatinine clearance in mL/min} = \frac{(140 - 65) \times 80 \times 1.23}{98}$$

$$= \frac{7380}{98}$$

$$= 75.31$$

75 mL/min to nearest whole number.

385 47.3 mL/min

BMI = weight (kg) ÷ height (m2)
= 88kg ÷ 2.81
= 31.3 kg/m2
BMI >30 therefore must use IBW
IBW = 50 + (2.3 × 6) = 63.8kg
Using the Cockcroft-Gault formula

$$\frac{(140 - 58) \times 63.8 \times 1.23}{136} = \frac{6434.87}{136} = 47.32$$

CrCl = 47.32 = 47.3 mL/min (rounded to one decimal place)

386 2640min

4,480mg/L = 0 hours;
2,240mg/L = 4 hours;
1,120mg/L = 8 hours;
560mg/L = 12 hours;
280mg/L = 16 hours;

140mg/L = 20 hours;
70mg/L = 24 hours;
35mg/L = 28 hours;
17.5mg/L = 32 hours;
8.75mg/L = 36 hours;
4.375mg/L = 40 hours;
2.1875mg/L (2,187.5 microgram/L) = 44 hours
44 hours × 60 mins = 2640 minutes.

387 15.6mg/L

0hrs = 1,000 mg/L;
3hrs = 500 mg/L;
6hrs = 250 mg/L;
9 hrs = 125 mg/L;
12 hrs = 62.5 mg/L;
15 hrs = 31.25 mg/L;
18 hrs = 15.62 mg/L = 15.6 mg/L (1 decimal place).

388 30.5mL

100mg tabs = 92mg suspension;
200mg = 184 mg oral suspension
Available as 30mg/5mL suspension:
 184 ÷ 30 × 5 = 30.667 mL per dose
Graduated syringe available as 0.5mL therefore rounded to 30.5mL per dose.

389 1 bottle

250 mcg tablet is equivalent to 200 mcg of elixr
Available as 50mcg per 1mL;
200 micrograms per 4mL;
4mL x 14 days = 56mL
Each bottle contains 60mL, therefore 1 bottle needed on discharge.

390 35%w/v

450mL – 250mL = 200mL (left of glucose 50%);
50g/100mL of glucose 50% w/v = 100g/200mL of glucose 50% w/v;
20g/100mL of glucose 20%w/v = 40g/200mL of glucose 20%w/v;

(100g + 40g) / (200mL + 200mL) (add weight and volume);
140g/400mL (Remember w/v is always per 100mL);
35g/100mL = 35%w/v (per 100mL).

391 **12mg/mL**

Displacement volume:

0.5mL/250mg, so 2mL displaced in 1g vial; 8 mL is added to the vial to reconstitute; therefore 8 mL + 2mL = 10mL of total volume

250 mg powder for solution for injection contains 30 mg of drug, therefore, 1g contains 120 mg of drug; 120mg/10mL = 12mg/mL.

Case based discussion answers

392 Consider travel health advice, will malaria prophylaxis be required, is it OTC or will it need to be on prescription, any general travel advice, any immunisations required? Any areas of high risk?
https://bnf.nice.org.uk/treatment-summaries/malaria-prophylaxis/
https://cks.nice.org.uk/topics/malaria-prophylaxis/
https://cks.nice.org.uk/topics/immunizations-travel/

393 Consider smoking status, consider cycle of change, consider any previous therapies, patients preferred route? Any night-time symptoms?
https://cks.nice.org.uk/topics/smoking-cessation/
https://www.nhs.uk/better-health/quit-smoking/
https://www.nhs.uk/live-well/quit-smoking/nhs-stop-smoking-services-help-you-quit/
https://www.ncsct.co.uk/

394 Consider any regular contraception, any risk of STI, any previous emergency hormonal contraception, is there any chance she is already pregnant? Consider options for patient, oral vs IUD? Consider timing of UPSI. Is the patient breastfeeding? Any other medication which may interact? High BMI? Cfounselling after issuing an oral medication.
https://cks.nice.org.uk/topics/contraception-emergency/
https://cks.nice.org.uk/topics/contraception-assessment/management/assessment-for-contraception/
https://cks.nice.org.uk/specialities/sexual-health/
https://bnf.nice.org.uk/interactions/

395 Consider timings of dose, compliance, other medication, INR monitoring, alcohol, diet, other healthcare professionals, risk of bleed?

https://cks.nice.org.uk/topics/atrial-fibrillation/
https://bnf.nice.org.uk/treatment-summaries/arrhythmias/
https://www.nhs.uk/conditions/atrial-fibrillation/

396 Consider options available, method of removing headlice, licensed OTC preps, any other medical conditions, tried anything in the past?
https://cks.nice.org.uk/topics/head-lice/
https://www.nhs.uk/conditions/head-lice-and-nits/

397 Under the Health Protection (Notification) Regulations 2010, registered medical practitioners (RMPs) have a statutory duty to notify the 'proper officer' at their local council, or local health protection team (HPT), of suspected cases of certain infectious diseases via a notification form.

Diseases notifiable to local authority proper officers include: Acute encephalitis; Acute infectious hepatitis; Acute meningitis; Acute poliomyelitis; Anthrax; Botulism; Brucellosis; Cholera; COVID-19; Diphtheria; Enteric fever (typhoid or paratyphoid fever); Food poisoning; Haemolytic uraemic syndrome (HUS); Infectious bloody diarrhoea; Invasive group A streptococcal disease; Legionnaires' disease; Leprosy; Malaria; Measles; Meningococcal septicaemia; Monkeypox; Mumps; Plague; Rabies; Rubella; Severe Acute Respiratory Syndrome (SARS); Scarlet fever; Smallpox; Tetanus; Tuberculosis; Typhus; Viral haemorrhagic fever (VHF); Whooping cough; Yellow fever. Consider why these diseases are notifiable.
https://www.gov.uk/guidance/notifiable-diseases-and-causative-organisms-how-to-report

398 Consider what information has been shared, who has to be notified, what actions need to be taken with your colleague and who should undertake them. What actions you need to take and what professional standards you need to adhere to.
https://digital.nhs.uk/services/national-data-opt-out/understanding-the-national-data-opt-out/confidential-patient-information
https://www.gov.uk/government/publications/accessing-ukhsa-protected-data/approval-standards-and-guidelines-confidential-patient-information
https://www.gov.uk/data-protection AND *https://www.rpharms.com/recognition/setting-professional-standards*

399 Part I: Review recent POM to P desogestrel switch, consider indications, contra-indications, when you can supply.
https://www.rpharms.com/resources/pharmacy-guides/desogestrel-p-medicine AND https://bnf.nice.org.uk/drugs/desogestrel/
https://www.gov.uk/government/consultations/hana-75-microgram-film-coated-tablets-desogestrel-public-consultation/public-feedback/a-public-consultation-on-reclassifying-two-medicines-containing-desogestrel-from-prescription-only-pom-to-pharmacy-p

399 Part II: Review recent POM to P estradiol switch, consider indications, contra-indications, when you can supply.
https://www.rpharms.com/resources/pharmacy-guides/estradiol-p-medicine AND https://bnf.nice.org.uk/drugs/estradiol/
https://www.gov.uk/government/consultations/consultation-on-proposal-to-make-gina-10-microgram-vaginal-tablets-estradiol-available-from-pharmacies#:~:text=A%20consultation%20document%20which%20summarises,who%20have%20not%20had%20a

400 Review MEP Chapter 4. The Responsible Pharmacist
https://www.rpharms.com/mep/4-the-responsible-pharmacist#gsc.tab=0

Index

A

abscess 14
acarbose 23
acebutolol 122
ACE inhibitors 39, 115
acetylcholine 129, 158, 162
aciclovir 102, 173
acne vulgaris 20
acromegaly 24
adalimumab 150, 151
Adcal D3 tablets 33
Addison's disease 42
adrenaline 57
adrenocortical insufficiency 78
adverse drug reactions 7
agranulocytosis 1, 43, 61, 130, 136, 152
akathisia 157
albuminuria 43
alcohol 122
alcohol dependence 69
alcohol use 14
alendronic acid 66, 131
alendronic acid tablets 33
alimemazine 57, 147
allopurinol 36, 75, 76, 160
alpha2-adrenoreceptor antagonists 50
alverine 152
alverine citrate 60, 148
aminoglycosides 141
aminosalicylates 152
amiodarone 12, 51, 142
amisulpride 3, 114
amitriptyline 4, 28, 47, 50, 60, 70, 73, 87, 149, 158
amlodipine 3, 5, 8, 10, 11, 12, 21, 23, 25, 39, 43, 51, 62, 63, 106, 115, 116, 119, 120, 134, 151
amorolfine 96, 174
amoxicillin 18, 35, 45, 46, 51, 63, 92, 100, 137, 151, 153, 180
anaemia 69, 100, 155
anakinra 75, 160
anaphylactic shock 77
anaphylaxis 34, 57
andexanet alfa IV 61
androgen deprivation therapy 74, 159
androgenetic alopecia 133
angina 7, 9, 39, 117, 122
antibacterial therapy 73
anticholinergics 129
antidepressant medications 50
antiepileptic drugs 1, 19
antiepileptic hypersensitivity syndrome 112
antifungal medications 45
antihistamines 57, 147
antihypertensive drugs 5
antimuscarinic drugs 148, 158
antipsychotic drugs 3, 4, 5, 6, 113, 138
anxiety disorder 47, 49
apixaban 44, 105
apraclonidine 76, 161
aripiprazole 3, 113, 114
aromatase inhibitors 159
arrythmias 135
arthritis 155, 156
aspirin 7, 9, 11, 16, 18, 24, 38, 39, 43, 73, 118, 134, 136, 151, 152
asthma 1, 16, 23, 40, 41, 47, 71, 72, 75, 87, 135, 157, 169
atenolol 11, 15, 16
atopic eczema 70, 155
atorvastatin 4, 5, 8, 9, 10, 11, 12, 39, 43, 63, 81, 136, 151
atrial fibrillation 6, 9, 29, 43, 52, 104, 141

atrophic vaginitis 46
atypical humerus fracture 23
autoimmune disease 108
avanafil 37
azathioprine 62, 66, 70, 150, 156
azithromycin 12, 51, 71, 90

B

bacterial conjunctivitis 73, 91, 94, 131, 171, 173
bacterial vaginosis 13, 46, 138
balslazine 62, 63
BCG vaccine 90
beclometasone 72, 92, 135, 157
beclomethasone 1, 2
beclomethasone dipropionate 56, 146
Bell's palsy 97
bendroflumethiazide 5, 11
benign prostatic hyperplasia 37
benzoyl peroxide 20, 124
benzydamine 32, 92, 171
benzyl benzoate 80, 164
benzylpenicillin 101, 102
beta2 agonists 135
Beta2 receptor agonists 41
beta-blockers 11, 16, 120, 123, 128, 134, 150, 161, 163
betamethasone 78, 162
bezafibrate 16, 122
bicalutamide 159
bimatoprost 76, 161
bipolar disorder 5, 17, 48, 139
bisacodyl 68
bisoprolol 7, 16, 18, 24, 25, 28, 40, 43, 44, 106, 134, 136
bisphosphonates 126, 151, 152, 159
black triangle scheme 82
black triangle symbol 166
bladder cancer 164, 165
bleomycin 9
blepharitis 91, 171
Blistex 94, 173

blood dyscrasias 155
body surface area formula 103, 104
bone marrow suppression 24, 158
Bonjela 94, 173
botulinum 78, 162
bradycardia 123
breast cancer 9, 74, 114, 159
brimonidine 76
brimonidine tartrate 161
brivaracetam 19
bromocriptine 24, 113
budesonide 40, 62
buprenorphine 18, 123

C

calamine lotion 87
calcium channel blocker 11
canagliflozin 52, 118, 143
candersartan 11
candida albicans 38
carbamazepine 1, 19, 28, 112, 124, 128
carbimazole 28, 32, 42, 130, 136
carbomer 76, 160
carbonic anhydrase inhibitor 161
cardiac dysfunction 74
cardiogenic shock 163
cardiomyocyte injury 119
carmellose 76
carmellose sodium 160
Carmex 94, 173
C. botulinum 162
C. difficile 19, 46, 124, 138
cefalexin 12, 13, 34, 35, 153
cefotaxime 121
ceftaroline 13
ceftazidime 13, 103
ceftriaxone 13, 121
celiprolol hydrochloride 122
cellulitis 17, 51, 141
cerfuroxime 13
certolizumab pegol 77, 161
ceterizine 57, 147

CHD 114, 115
chemotherapy 9, 154
chickenpox 33, 87, 88, 169
chlamydia 46, 90, 170
chloramphenicol 33, 93, 94, 173
chlormethiazole 99
chlorphenamine 28, 57, 66, 87, 147
cholestatic jaundice 51
ciclosporin 15, 70, 122
cimetidine 65, 67
Cimzia 161
ciprofloxacin 14, 18, 19, 44, 45, 51, 59, 123, 141
cirrhosis 61, 149
citalopram 4, 5, 15, 17, 26, 27, 115, 123, 128
clarithromycin 13, 14, 35, 44, 45, 63, 121, 132, 151
Clenil 41, 58, 71, 135
clindamycin 19, 66, 153
clobazam 19, 28
clobetasone 95, 172
clobetasone butyrate 93
clonazepam 28
clopidogrel 9, 11, 16, 43, 51, 61, 63, 64, 118, 136, 141, 149, 151
clotrimazole 20, 37, 38, 46, 55, 86, 93, 96, 134, 175
clozapine 4, 114
co-amoxiclav 2, 13, 14, 98, 120, 121
co-beneldopa 30, 129
co-careldopa 2, 3
Cockcroft-Gault formula 101, 102, 108, 187
co-codamol 101
co-danthramer 55, 145
co-danthrusate 145
codeine 66, 67
co-dydramol 68
colchicine 75, 160
colecalciferol 21, 22, 42, 69, 106, 155
colon cancer 68

constipation 55, 56, 60, 67, 68, 78, 129, 145, 158, 163
contact dermatitis 33
controlled drugs 85
convulsions 141
COPD 34, 41, 72, 100, 157
Corminaty 77
corticosteroids 78, 131, 152, 160, 162
COVID-19 vaccination 77
COVID-19 vaccine 90, 161
CRB-65 137
Crohn's disease 35, 56, 62, 63, 64, 70, 146, 150, 151, 156
crotamiton 80, 164
Cushing's Syndrome 126
cyanocobalamin 25
cyclizine 57, 147
cyclophosphamide 9
cyproterone acetate 159
cystitis 71
cytarabine 74
cytotoxic drugs 158

D

Daktacort 168
dalteparin sodium 7, 8, 118
dantrolene 113
dapagliflozin 7, 23, 118
daunorubicin 118
dementia 49
denosumab 159
depression 1, 4, 15, 18, 49, 138
dermatitis 172
desogestrel 36, 132, 192
dexamethasone 78, 106, 162
diabetes mellitus 3, 7, 8, 13, 21, 22, 23, 31, 41, 43, 45, 53, 75, 80, 81, 130, 135, 142, 160, 168
diabetic ketoacidosis 118, 143
diarrhoea 7, 17, 40, 43, 45, 47, 66, 137, 149, 153
diazepam 4, 5, 47, 86, 98, 177

diclofenac 17, 29, 30, 123, 129
digoxin 12, 39, 43, 51, 103, 104, 109, 120, 141, 152, 182
digoxin toxicity 58, 148
dihydrotestosterone 144
diltiazem 12, 40, 51, 119
dipyridamole 9, 118
disulfiram 61
diuretics 115
diverticulitis 13
dizziness 61
DMARD therapy 70
docusate sodium 55, 66, 79, 145
dopamine 113, 114
dorzolamide 77, 161
doxazosin 5, 70, 99, 116
doxorubicin 9, 118
doxycycline 13, 18, 35, 44, 45, 46, 51, 59, 67, 121
dry eye 76, 91, 171
dulaglutide 52, 142
DVLA 1
dysmenorrhoea 153
dysuria 20, 67

E

Earcalm 92
echocardiogram 119
eczema 95, 174
EEA prescribers 167
ejection fraction 7
EllaOne 91
emergency hormonal contraception 190
empagliflozin 22, 23, 31, 118, 126, 130
enalapril 11, 38, 120
endocarditis 10
enteropathy 74, 159
epilepsy 18, 82, 107, 139, 165
epirubicin 118
erectile dysfunction 23
escitalopram 15, 27, 128
Estraderm Mx patch 36

estradiol 36, 59, 133, 177, 192
estriol 133
ethinylestradiol 36, 133
ethosuximide 19
ethylene glycol 145
etonogestrel implant 36
etoposide 74, 103, 182, 183
exotoxins 162

F

familial hyperlipidaemia 61
famotidine 61, 63, 66, 151
febuxostat 75, 160
felodipine 12, 24
fentanyl 77, 86
ferinject 69
ferric carboxymaltose 59, 148
ferric derisomaltose 148
ferrous fumarate 59
ferrous gluconate 59
ferrous iron 100
ferrous sulfate 59, 100
ferrous sulphate 42, 59, 69, 154
fidaxomicin 19, 124
finasteride 37, 54, 70, 144, 156
flucloxacillin 10, 13, 17, 18, 51, 59, 120, 141
fluconazole 20, 37, 38, 45, 46, 96, 134, 137, 174
fludrocortisone 78, 162
fluoxetine 5, 15, 36, 50, 140
flupenthixol decanoate 4
fluticasone 14, 23, 56, 78, 146, 147
Flutiform 57
fluvastatin 12, 120
folate 21
folate levels 22
folic acid 15, 42, 58, 69, 154, 155
folic acid antagonist 70
formoterol 57, 146
formoterol fumarate 56, 146
fostair 75
Fragmin 118

Fraser guidelines 80, 163, 164
furosemide 17, 25, 39, 40, 43, 44, 52, 98, 142
fusidic acid 33

G

gabapentin 36
galactorrhoea 3, 113
gastric ulcer 64
gastroenteritis 35
gastrointestinal bleeding 61, 66
gastrointestinal ulcers 117
gastro-oesophageal reflux disease 61
Gaviscon 65, 67
gemcitabine 9
gentamicin 10, 13, 14, 51, 59, 121, 141
Gillick competency 80, 164
glaucoma 23, 76
gliclazide 22, 23, 24, 31, 41, 125, 130
glimepiride 52, 106
GLP-1 receptor agonists 53, 142
glucagon 79, 163
glucocorticoid 162
glucocorticoid receptor agonists 41
glucosamine 33
glucose 99, 121, 160, 188
glucotabs 31
glyceryl trinitrate 40
glycopyrronium bromide 56, 146
goserelin 75, 159
gout 75, 160
GRACE 117
grapefruit juice 15
gynaecomastia 74, 159

H

haloperidol 3
HAS-BLED 116
headache 43
headlice 110, 191
heart failure 6, 23, 44, 52, 103, 119, 125, 142, 159

hepatic encephalopathy 56, 145
hepatitis 51, 141
hepatitis A vaccine 90
hepatitis B vaccine 90
hepatitis C vaccine 90
hepatotoxicity 155
herpes simplex 33, 102, 173
HIV infection 125
Hodgkin lymphoma 104
hormonal contraception 80, 91, 110, 133
hormone replacement therapy 111
H-Pylori 35, 63, 131, 132
humulin M3 31
hydrocortisone 42, 86, 93, 95, 96, 172, 174
hydroxocobalamin 69, 155
hydroxypropyl guar 160
hyoscine butylbromide 68, 154
hyoscine hydrobromide 114
hyperactivity 28
hypercalcaemia 47, 58, 148
hypercholesterolaemia 21
hyperglycaemia 47, 138
hyperkalaemia 15, 43, 47, 58, 122
hyperlipidemia 38
hypermagnesaemia 58
hypernatraemia 59
hyperprolactinaemia 3, 113, 114
hypersalivation 28, 114
hypertension 4, 7, 8, 9, 10, 11, 16, 21, 23, 25, 39, 40, 47, 49, 71, 87, 115, 120, 127, 149, 156
hyperthermia 113
hyperthyroidism 136
hypocalcaemia 48, 58, 148
hypoglycaemia 31, 43, 130
hypokalaemia 48, 58, 72, 107, 148, 157
hypokalemia 40
hypomagnaesemia 148
hypomagnaseia 48
hypomagnesaemia 59, 152
hyponatraemia 58, 59, 148

hypoparathyroidism 148
hypotension 24, 119, 120, 126
hypothyroidism 25, 32, 41, 76, 116, 127, 135
hypromellose 76, 160

I

ibuprofen 15, 21, 79, 87, 162, 163, 169
idarubicin 119
immunosuppressant medication 70, 155
impetigo 33, 88, 131, 169
impulse control disorders 113
inclisiran 61
indacaterol 56
indapamide 43
infliximab 62, 63, 70, 150, 151, 156
influenza vaccine 90
insomnia 48, 139
insulin glargine 41, 52
interleukin-1 inhibitors 160
intra-uterine contraceptive device 36
ipratropium 40, 41, 72, 135
iron 49
irritable bowel syndrome 60, 66, 68, 145, 148, 149, 152, 154
ischaemic heart disease 16
isoniazid 20, 21
isosorbide dinitrate 16
isosorbide mononitrate 7, 18, 122
isphaghula husk 55, 60, 145, 148
itraconazole 45, 46

J

jaundice 141

K

Kawasaki disease 107
keratitis 73, 91
ketamine 77
ketoacidosis 7, 74
ketoconazole 45, 46, 86, 93, 172

L

labetalol 11, 16, 120
lacosamide 112
lactic acidosis 32, 125
lactulose 55, 60, 68, 79, 145, 146, 148
lamotrigine 112
lansoprazole 32, 35, 59, 61, 63, 65, 67, 68, 75, 106, 151, 152, 153
latanoprost 161
laxatives 55, 56, 145, 146, 148, 149, 154
Laxido 107
letrozole 75, 159
leukotriene receptor antagonists 41, 147, 157
levetiracetam 1, 19, 107
levobunolol 77
levobunolol hydrochloride 161
levodopa 30, 129
Levonelle 91
levonorgestrel 36, 132, 133
levothyroxine 25, 32, 42, 64, 76, 116, 135
lidocaine 100, 180
linaclotide 55, 60, 145, 149
linagliptin 21, 22, 23, 31, 41, 130
liraglutide 23, 60
lisinopril 16, 106
lithium 5, 6, 17, 48, 49, 50, 115, 116, 123, 139, 140
liver dysfunction 128
liver failure 61, 74
liver function tests 22
liver toxicity 126
lofepramine 4, 47, 115
loperamide 17, 60, 149
loratadine 17, 57, 147
lorazepam 47, 83, 166
losartan 5, 11, 18
lymecycline 44, 51
lymphadenopathy 1

M

macrogol 55, 79, 145, 163
Madopar 30
magnesium 49, 65
magnesium sulphate 105
magnesium trisilicate 66
malaria 190
malathion 80, 164
mania 165
measles 88
mebendazole 24, 95, 96, 175
mebeverine 152
mebeverine hydrochloride 60
megaloblastic anaemia 154
melatonin 24, 129
melphalan 73, 158
MenB vaccine 90
meningioma 74, 159
meningitis 13
menstruation 36
mercaptopurine 70, 150, 156
mesalazine 64, 68, 152, 154
metaprolol 128
metformin 3, 7, 9, 21, 22, 23, 31, 41, 52, 73, 75, 81, 106, 125, 130, 135, 142
methadone 4, 5, 115
methocarbamol 24
methotrexate 21, 24, 63, 70, 74, 126, 150, 155, 156
methyldopa 11, 24
methylnaltrexone bromide 55
methylphenidate 47
methylprednisolone 25, 78, 126, 162
metoclopramide 29, 68
metoprolol 39
metronidazole 13, 14, 35, 37, 38, 45, 46, 59, 63, 121, 122, 132, 133, 134, 138, 148, 151
MHRA 166
miconazole 45, 46, 86, 96, 137, 175
Microgynon 54, 91, 144
migraine 26, 28, 29, 48, 54, 82, 124, 165, 168
mineralcorticoid 162
mirabegron 70, 156
mirtazapine 2, 4, 47, 50, 64, 73, 115, 140
misoprostol 65
mitomycin 74
mometasone 78
mometasone furoate 56, 93, 162, 172
monoarthritis 77
monoclonal antibodies 70
montelukast 40, 41, 57, 71, 72, 147, 157
morphine 86
morphine sulfate 84, 167
mouth ulcers 7, 21
multiple myeloma 73
muscarinic receptor antagonists 41, 135
myasthenia gravis 14
mycophenolate 21, 70, 155
myelosuppression 70, 150, 156
myocardial infarction 4, 6, 11, 15, 18, 100, 122
myopathy 122

N

nadolol 150
naloxegol 68, 154
naproxen 15, 18, 32, 33, 36, 67, 68, 75, 153
nefopam 17
nephrotoxicity 45, 51, 141
neural tube defects 58
neuroleptic malignant syndrome 113
neuropathic pain 30
neuropathy 124
neutropenia 130, 155
nicorandil 7, 117
nicotine replacement therapy 110
nifedipine 12, 21, 40, 43, 120
nightmares 28
nitrofurantoin 44, 46, 67, 97, 137, 153, 176

norethisterone 36, 132
notifiable diseases' 110
novorapid insulin vials 31
NSAIDs 151, 152, 153, 160
NSTEMI 43, 117, 119
number needed to harm 105
Nurofen 87, 169
NYHA 117

O

obesity 149
oedema 142
oesophageal varices 62
oesopharyngeal varices 61
oestrogen 82
olanzapine 3, 29, 114
omeprazole 9, 16, 63, 66, 106
ondansetron 4, 5, 68, 115, 154
oral candidiasis 40, 135
Oramorph 100
ORBIT 116
organ rejection 155
orlistat 86
osteoporosis 66, 74, 126, 131, 136, 153, 159
otitis media 13
Otomize 92
ototoxicity 51, 141
ovarian cancer 103
oxcarbazepine 112
oxprenolol hydrochloride 122
oxybutynin 65, 71, 156
oxycodone 17, 18, 86, 168
oxytetracycline 18
ozempic 52, 142

P

palliative care 29, 47, 129
Panadol 87
pantoprazole 19, 62
paracetamol 2, 8, 10, 14, 17, 18, 20, 22, 24, 25, 26, 27, 32, 33, 45, 59, 74, 78, 87, 90, 162, 169

paraesthesia 21, 148
paraffin 160, 161
Paramol 87
parecoxib 77
Parkinson's disease 2, 30, 113
paroxetine 15, 47, 50, 140
penicillin 13, 34, 35, 132, 137, 151, 166
peppermint oil 60, 66, 152
peptic ulcer 151
perioperative anaphylactic reaction 162
peripheral neuropathy 74
peripheral oedema 134
peritonsillar abscess 171
permethrin 80, 93, 164, 172
pertuzumab 75
phenobarbital 112
phenoxymethylpenicillin 83
phenytoin 109, 112
pheonxymethylpenicillin 92
phosphodiesterase type-4 inhibitors 72, 157
pindolol 16, 122
pioglitazone 7, 23, 31, 41, 52, 81, 125, 126, 142, 164, 165
pneumococcal vaccine 90
pneumococcus 170
pneumonia 13
polycystic ovary syndrom 31
polyvinyl alcohol 160
POM register 85
postural hypotension 61
potassium 44, 49, 136, 152
potassium chloride 107, 151
potassium permanganate 104
pravastatin 12
prednisolone 14, 40, 41, 63, 64, 70, 71, 72, 75, 78, 97, 100, 106, 151, 160, 162
pregabalin 30, 84, 129, 167
Pregnancy Prevention Programme 26, 127, 165, 167
primary dysmenorrhea 67
primidone 8, 112

procyclidine hydrochloride 3
progesterone 36, 132
progestogen 82
prolactin 113, 114
promethazine 27, 147
propofol 77
propranolol 11, 16, 28, 62, 79, 128, 150
propylthiouracil 42
prostaglandin 161
prostaglandin analogue 76
prostate cancer 8, 74
prostatic hyperplasia 71, 156, 175
proton pump inhibitors 152
psoriasis 47
psychosis 47
pulmonary embolism 8
purines 160
pyelonephritis 8, 98, 124
pyrexia 44
pyridoxine 20, 21, 124

Q

QRISK3 117
QT interval prolongation 5, 17, 123, 128
quinolones 123, 141

R

rabies vaccine 90
radiotherapy 74, 154
ramipril 4, 5, 9, 10, 11, 15, 26, 27, 39, 43, 62, 83, 115, 119, 122, 127, 134, 136
renal failure 74
renal function 127
Replens 37, 133
responsible pharmacist role 111
revalidation records 89
rhabdomyolysis 14, 122, 132, 151
rheumatoid arthritis 68, 70
rifampicin 10, 14, 83, 119
rifaximin 83, 166
riluzole 83
risedronate 24, 126

risk scoring systems 6, 7
CHA2DS2-VASc 6
GRACE 6
HAS-BLED 6
NEWS2 6
NYHA 6
ORBIT 6
QRISK3 6
risperidone 3, 114
ritonavir 21, 125
rivaroxaban 10, 15, 43, 119
rizatriptan 83
roflumilast 72, 157
rosuvastatin 12, 15
rotigotine 2, 3, 113
rubella 169
rufinamide 112

S

salbutamol 2, 16, 23, 40, 41, 56, 57, 71, 72, 87, 135, 146, 157
salicylic acid 86
salmeterol 40, 56, 57, 71, 135, 147
Sando-K 65
Saxenda 149
scabies 33, 80, 93, 164
scarlet fever 88
schizophrenia 4, 48
scleritis 91
seborrhoeic dermatitis 93
Seebri Breezhaler 56
semaglutide 3, 7, 22, 81
senna 55, 60, 145, 146
sepsis 173
Seretide Accuhaler 57
sertraline 4, 15, 18, 47, 50, 59, 114, 122, 123, 138, 140, 148
SGLT-2 inhibitors 118, 143
shingles 88
sildenafil 37, 54
simvastatin 10, 12, 14, 22, 36, 39, 119, 122, 132, 134

sinusitis 78, 162
sitagliptin 52
SNRIs 138
sodium 44, 50, 59, 98, 101, 181
sodium chloride 107, 121
sodium cromoglycate 93
sodium hyaluronate 76, 160
sodium valproate 1, 26, 81, 84, 85, 105, 127, 165
solifenacin 59, 71
Solpadeine 87
spacer devices 57
spironolactone 26, 44, 52, 62, 136
SSRIs 15, 50, 114, 140, 151, 152
Standards for Pharmacy Professionals 82
STEMI 39, 134
St John's Wort 2
stroke 109
subconjunctival haemorrhage 73, 91, 171
Sudafed 96
sulfasalazine 70, 73
sulphonylureas 125, 130
sulpiride 114
sumatriptan 48, 87, 96, 139, 168
suxamethonium 77, 162
sympatomimetics 161

T

tacrolimus 70, 99, 155
tadalafil 37, 54, 133
tafluprost 161
tamoxifen 75, 159
tamsulosin 54, 71, 96, 156, 175
tardive dyskinesia 114
temocillin 8
tendonitis 45, 123
terazosin 54
terbinafine 45, 46, 86, 93
terbutaline 15
terlipressin 62, 149

testosterone 144
tetracyline 35
TFN-a inhibitors 161
theobroma oil 98, 105, 184
theophylline 40, 72, 100, 157
thiamine 61, 69, 154
thiazide 120
thiopurine methyltransferase 150
threadworms 95, 175
thrombocytopenia 1
thyroxine 130
ticagrelor 9, 118
timolol 28
tinzaparin 16, 107
tioguanine 150
tiotropium 72, 157
tonic-clonic seizure 1
topiramate 28
tramadol 2, 14, 17, 18, 21, 64, 84, 112, 167
tranexamic acid PO 62
transient ischaemic attack 9, 15, 52, 61
trastuzumab 74, 159
travellers diarrhoea 35
travoprost 161
trazodone 50, 140
Trelegy Ellipta 57
triamcinolone 162
tricyclic antidepressants 114, 115
trifluoperazine 3, 114
Trimbow 57
trimethoprim 46, 51, 67, 71, 157
tuberculosis 20, 90, 170
tumour flare 74

U

ulcerative colitis 64, 68, 106, 146
umeclidinium bromide 56, 146
undecylenic acid 86
urea 44
uric acid 160
urinary disorders 126

urinary incontinence 59, 152
urinary symptoms 70, 71
urinary tract infection 44, 67, 153, 157
uveitis 73, 91, 158

V

vaginal atrophy 133
vaginal candidiasis 46, 174
vaginal thrush 55
valproic acid 3
vancomycin 46, 108, 138
vardenafil 37, 54
vedolizumab 63, 150
venlafaxine 4, 47, 50, 115, 138
venous thromboembolism 8, 133
Ventolin Evohaler 56
ventricular arrhythmia 115
verapamil 10, 12, 62, 119, 120
verruca 86
veterinary medicines 85
Vigabatrin 1
vilanterol 56, 146

vincristine 74, 159
viral conjunctivitis 73, 91
vitamin B 69
vitamin B12 22, 69, 125
vitamin D deficiency 69, 155
vulvovaginal candidasis 38, 134

W

warfarin 43, 52, 110, 136
Wernicke's encephalopathy 69, 154

X

xanthine-oxidase inhibitors 160

Z

zinc 22, 50
zinc undecylenate 86
zoledronic acid 75, 159
zolpidem 48, 139
Zonisamide 1
zopiclone 27
Zovirax 94, 173